T0144419

BASIC HEALTH PUBLICATIONS USER'S GUIDE

TO ANTI-AGING NUTRIENTS

Discover How You Can Slow Down the Aging Process and Increase Energy.

JACK CHALLEM AND ROSE-MARIE GIONTA ALFIERI, M.A.

JACK CHALLEM Series Editor

The information contained in this book is based upon the research and personal and professional experiences of the authors. It is not intended as a substitute for consulting with your physician or other healthcare provider. Any attempt to diagnose and treat an illness should be done under the direction of a healthcare professional.

The publisher does not advocate the use of any particular healthcare protocol but believes the information in this book should be available to the public. The publisher and authors are not responsible for any adverse effects or consequences resulting from the use of the suggestions, preparations, or procedures discussed in this book. Should the reader have any questions concerning the appropriateness of any procedures or preparations mentioned, the authors and the publisher strongly suggest consulting a professional healthcare advisor.

Series Editor: Jack Challem
Editor: Stephany Evans
Typesetter: Gary A. Rosenberg
Series Cover Designer: Mike Stromberg

Basic Health Publications User's Guides are published by Basic Health Publications, Inc.

CONTENTS

INTRODUCTION

One of the least pleasant facts of life is that as long as we are alive we will age. Old Man Time is an equal opportunity nemesis, and not one of us can outrun him or escape him. Starting in our twenties, time begins to chip away at our health and fitness through the downward pull of gravity, environmental damage, old-fashioned wear and tear, cellular changes in our bodies, and through the effects of lifestyle choices. That is a simple, unchangeable reality.

Aging is not a single condition. It can most accurately be defined as the accumulation of those time-related changes that lead eventually to disease and death. Its varied effects are felt from middle age (roughly, age forty to age sixty). Decreased energy and sexual drive, digestive troubles, memory deterioration, wrinkles, thinning skin, muscle atrophy, and assorted diseases, such as heart disease or diabetes, are some of the most common.

While none of us can permanently stop the ticking clock of our lives, is there anything we can do to forestall or alleviate some of these age-related conditions? Is it possible to prevent some of the damaging effects of aging in order to slow down the process, and to enjoy greater energy and health well into our middle and later years?

The answer to both of these questions is yes. Increasingly, scientific evidence suggests that while we may not be able to stop the aging process, it is possible to prevent many of the diseases associated with aging and to slow the rate at which our bodies age. Numerous studies have identified several nutritional supplements that can reverse or prevent the damage to our cells that not only ages us in appearance, but also increases our risk for several age-related diseases, including diabetes, Alzheimer's disease, heart disease, and cancer.

Many of these supplements, which will be presented in this book, are antioxidants. These groups of vitamins, minerals, and enzymes are extremely important for anti-aging because they help to protect the body against free-radical damage. Free radicals are atoms that contain unpaired electrons. They damage cells in an organism by stealing electrons in an effort to become stable. This damage causes many of the undesirable and unhealthy effects of aging. The free-radical theory of aging is discussed more fully in Chapter 1.

This book also delves into lifestyle issues, such as diet, exercise, and unhealthy habits, all of which contribute to how we age. This is one area that, unlike our genetic makeup, is entirely within our control. Making simple changes in these areas of your life can work wonders in helping you to lead a youthful life—whatever your age. You may have a biological age of sixty, but with a combination of healthy lifestyle habits and supplementation with nutrients, your actual age in terms of vitality and risk for disease may be far younger.

According to the National Center for Health Statistics, the life expectancy for Americans has reached an all-time high of nearly seventy-seven years, with an increase in people living into their nineties and even hundreds. It is no longer such a surprise to read about someone celebrating a

100th birthday. You have to ask yourself though, how healthy, how vital is the person? For most of us, it is desirable to live a long life, but how much better for that life to be full of good health and vitality! The *User's Guide to Anti-Aging Nutrients* will help you make choices about those nutrients that can enable you to live your youngest—and healthiest—at any age. Here's to being eighty years—or more—young!

CHAPTER 1

SOME BASICS ON THE QUESTION OF AGING

You've probably known people who at age fifty or even sixty have the glow, energy, and vibrancy of people in their early twenties. They just exude health and well-being, are active, embrace life with enthusiasm, and don't seem to be plagued by the usual age-related problems. Most likely, they are living lives that support energy production rather than depletion. There are so many factors that contribute to how well you will age. A major one of these is the amount and type of damage your cells have sustained due to free-radical production in your body throughout your life. In addition, there are particular lifestyle habits you may choose and maintain, which can either accelerate or slow the aging process. In this chapter, we'll explore these factors as well as some key ways you can put the brakes on aging.

Free Radicals Gone Amok

Free radicals occur in all living things. An atom, when it is stable, contains a balance of paired electrons, which encircle the nu - cleus. Free radicals are atoms or molecules in which at least one electron is unpaired, causing an instability. This instability causes

Free Radicals
Atoms with unpaired electrons that damage cells and cause aging.

the electrons to be very reactive—they can bond easily with other molecules and, in so doing, can cause damage through the process we know as oxidation.

The most common free radical in humans is an oxygen radical, which occurs in the mitochondria when an unpaired electron interacts with oxygen. Mitochondria are our cells' power plants, the tiny structures in our cells that provide energy in the chemical form of adenosine triphosphate (ATP). ATP provides the fuel for all of our life functions, helping our hearts to pump and our lungs to take in and distribute oxygen when we breathe. When free radicals are formed in the mitochondria, they reduce the power of the mitochondria to produce energy efficiently. Worse yet, they often damage DNA, as well as proteins and fats, inside the mitochondria.

According to the free-radical theory of aging, it is this damage that causes us to age and to become more vulnerable to certain diseases such as atherosclerosis (hardening of the arteries) and cancer. In addition, damage done by free radicals to collagen and elastin can cause our skin to thin and age.

And yet, free radicals do play an important role in maintaining good health. After all, they are created as a natural byproduct of oxidation, which occurs when the body uses oxygen and the nutrients from the foods we eat to create energy. Some free radicals work to fight disease; for example, those produced by the immune system are important for fighting viruses and bacteria. For such purposes, free radicals should be present in small numbers in our bodies. The problem occurs when these free radicals are produced in excess. In addition to being formed through the normal oxidation of nutrients, free radicals are created through exposure to radiation and pollutants, and through the breakdown of fat into energy, as in aerobic exercise.

Antioxidants to Sop up the Damage

Just as the body produces free radicals, it also has its own means of neutralizing them when there are too many or after their work is done. Our bodies produce free-radical scavengers in the form of certain enzymes. These enzymes attack and neutralize the free radicals. However, even with this built in clean-up crew, our bodies can be overwhelmed by excessive free radicals when under stress by environmental pollutants, poor dietary habits, or destructive habits, such as smoking or excessive alcohol consumption. Still, there are ways that we can reduce the number of potentially damaging free radicals in our bodies.

In addition to those scavengers that occur naturally in the body, several antioxidant nutrients, such as vitamins E and C, the hormone melatonin, and alpha-lipoic acid keep free-radical levels in check by attaching to the free electrons in a free radical and neutralizing it. The problem is that many of us do not consume an adequate amount of antioxidants through our diets alone. This is especially true as we age, when we need even more antioxidant activity because of the free radicals that have built up over the years.

Researchers have found that dietary supplementation with antioxidants may help to fight age-related diseases thought to be caused, at least in part, by an excess of free radicals. These diseases include atherosclerosis, cancer, and some neurodegenerative diseases. In the chapters to come, you will learn about several nutritional supplements that have strong scientific backing for their positive role in an anti-aging program.

Lifestyle Habits Play a Major Role

Before having a look at some of the individual promising anti-aging supplements, let's talk a little about lifestyle and how changes you make in the way you live your life can have dramatic effects on how you age. It is a fact that much illness, disability, and even death that is associated with the chronic diseases we tend to associate with aging are preventable. In fact, did you know that 40 percent of deaths in our country are attributed to smoking, being inactive, poor diet, or the misuse of alcohol? That's a huge percentage, and all of those factors are entirely within our control. The Centers for Disease Control and Prevention estimates that poor diet and physical inactivity alone lead to 300,000 deaths each year. Only smoking causes more deaths! Let's take a quick look at diet and activity.

The Importance of Diet

As we age, eating a healthful diet consisting of foods that are rich in nutrients, such as fruits and vegetables, and avoiding empty calories is vital. A healthy eating plan will keep your skin and hair vibrant and healthy, and will help prevent nutrition-related diseases such as heart disease, diabetes, and osteoporosis (thinning of the bone). Diet becomes increasingly important as you get older, because your ability to absorb nutrients declines with age, as does your body's ability to assimilate or use the nutrients that you take in.

In the United States, type II diabetes has reached epidemic status. You probably have read the numerous front-page articles published recently about this new health epidemic. Seventeen million Americans have diabetes and more than 200,000 die every year due to complications of the disease. Worse yet, people are being diagnosed at younger and younger ages, in their twenties and thirties, even in their teens—this was unheard of in the not so distant past. In fact, type II diabetes used to be called adult-onset diabetes because it was primarily diagnosed in people over age fifty. Not anymore.

Why is this epidemic occurring now? Because of our poor diets. Intake of too many unrefined carbohydrates, such as white flour and white bread, causes the blood to be flooded with glucose. This, in turn, forces the pancreas to work really hard to pump out more and more insulin to transport glucose from the blood to the cells. Eventually, a person can become what is known as insulin resistant, which means the insulin simply is no longer as effective against the blood sugar. And so, elevated glucose levels remain in the body, and that person is on the road to diabetes. Insulin resistance can lead to Syndrome X, a condition that puts you at greater risk for diabetes and heart disease.

Insulin Resistance
A condition characterized by the body's inability to effectively transport glucose from the blood.

Compounding the problem is the fact that when one's glucose level is above normal, glucose is oxidized readily, creating free radicals, which can then increase one's risk for heart disease. In addition, the process known as glycosylation (when glucose binds to proteins and cross-links them) is associated with aging and disease. Watching your food intake carefully, controlling your portion sizes, and making sure that you choose foods that are low in sugar, as well as low in saturated fat, can go a long way toward keeping you young.

You've Got to Move It

Denham Harman, M.D., Ph.D., of the University of Nebraska College of Medicine, is a major proponent of the free-radical theory of aging and is widely considered its founder. He has conducted several studies on free-radical involvement in aging. Dr. Harman recommends reducing caloric intake by 10 percent in order to decrease oxygen consumption and, therefore, cut the rate of production of free radicals in the body. But just cutting calories is not enough.

Traditionally, as we age, we tend to be less active. Today, however, even children are not as active as they were years ago, spending more time at their computers or in front of the television. The importance of being physically active for at least thirty minutes on most days of the week was the cornerstone of the 1996 *Report of the Surgeon General on Physical Activity and Health.* Physical activity was shown to protect people against age-related diseases such as heart disease, certain cancers, and osteoporosis. In addition, it was found to help relieve joint stiffness and to increase range of movement in people with arthritis. In October 2002, the *Journal of the American Medical Association* (JAMA) re - ported that exercise training may improve the cardiovascular health of people with type II diabetes and hypertension.

Weight and Life Expectancy

Proper diet and physical activity are two sides of the seesaw that keeps your weight at a healthy balance. Perhaps the most important reason to lead an active life is to prevent obesity, which is a risk factor for diabetes, high blood pressure, and heart disease. Like diabetes, which is more likely to be diagnosed in people who are overweight, obesity has become a national epidemic.

Recent research has shown just how unhealthy obesity is: A study reported in *JAMA* showed that if you are obese at age twenty, your life may be shortened by up to twenty years. This report was released one day after another study published in the *Annals of Internal Medicine* presented the results of a Dutch study on 3,400 middle-aged Americans in which the researchers discovered that being overweight at age forty can reduce life expectancy by three years.

Walking

A study on walking in postmenopausal women that was reported in the *Archives of Internal Medicine* looked at 229 women ten years after they participated in a clinical walking trial. The women who walked regularly reported fewer cases of heart disease, hospitalizations, surgeries, and falls compared with a control group of non-walkers.

Cardiovascular Fitness

The National Institute on Aging recommends thirty minutes of activity that makes you breathe harder on most or all days of the week to build stamina and increase cardiovascular fitness.

A study reported in *Circulation* indicated that when middle-aged men took part in a program of moderate exercise (one hour, four to five times per week), their cardiovascular fitness returned to levels comparable to a twenty year old. This study showed that as little as six months of moderate physical activity can indeed turn back time!

Muscle Tone

After age twenty, you lose as much as a half pound of muscle a year, so it is also important to incorporate training for your muscles (strength training) into your routine.

Muscle loss is due mostly to not using your muscles enough. It's the old use it or lose it phenomenon. Having enough muscle not only makes you look more defined and younger, but also helps you to perform activities of daily life (such as getting up and down) easily. Most experts recommend training with weights at least twice a week, for approximately twenty minutes each session. Finally, stretching and balance training, such as standing on one leg without holding on to anything, is also helpful as you age. If you are a man over age forty or woman over age fifty, make sure you check with your doctor before beginning a vigorous exercise program.

In *The American Council of Exercise Fit Facts* (2001), Dr. Benjamin Levine, a coauthor of the above study, states, "Starting an exercise program when you are older is still useful and can combat the effects of aging." Dr. Levine is associate professor of internal medicine and director of the Institute for Exercise and Environmental Medicine.

Unhealthy Habits Result in Unhealthy Skin

While gravity plays a role in the creation of wrinkles, much skin damage is the result of poor habits. Unfortunately, many of these habits date back to our youth. When we are young and can't even imagine aging, we may tend to take our fine young skin for granted. However, late nights out, fast food eating, sun worshiping, and binge drinking at age twenty can be the cause of our unnecessarily losing health and vitality. Their negative effects are cumulative.

Smoking

In addition to their potentially devastating effects on long-term health, drinking alcohol in excess and smoking cigarettes also wreak havoc with the skin. Cigarette smokers have more wrinkles than nonsmokers of the same age, complexion, and history of sun exposure. Scientists believe this is because smoking can damage fibers in the skin known as elastin, which give skin its resiliency, like a rubber band's ability to snap back.

Alcohol

Recently, there has been growing evidence that moderate alcohol consumption may benefit cardiovascular health. It appears that the antioxidants in alcohol, especially wine, help to keep blood vessels clear. While this may mean it makes sense for people without drinking problems to have a glass or two of wine with dinner, it in no way is an endorsement to go out and pound drinks at the local bar. If you do have a tendency to drink too much, it may be wiser to skip the alcohol entirely. While moderate alcohol use may be associated with a reduced risk of heart disease, overuse of alcohol is also associated with liver disease, highway fatalities, and other life-threatening conditions.

Sun

Finally, the National Institute on Aging advises that the simplest way to keep your skin young looking is to stay out of the sun. Sunlight, with its ultraviolet light, also damages elastin in the skin. As a result, your skin is unable to snap back after stretching and wrinkles form. Sun exposure also dries out the skin. If you are going to be out in the sun, be sure to use a sunblock with a sun protection factor (SPF) of at least 15, and try to avoid the sun during its strongest hours (from 11 A.M. to 2 P.M.).

CHAPTER 2

ACETYL-L-CARNITINE

The mitochondria—those small structures in your cells that produce energy—may be thought of as busy power plants, constantly at work to produce the energy the body needs. Through a series of chemical reactions within the mitochondria, glucose and fat are converted to adenosine triphosphate (ATP), the chemical form of energy. This is the energy that the body uses for the basic functions of life: to breathe, to keep the heart beating, and to think.

Because of their great level of chemical activity, the mitochondria are susceptible to damage by free radicals. Several recent studies indicate that certain nutrients enhance the activity of the mitochondria and are effective in combating the aging process. These nutrients help to prevent the accumulated damage to the mitochondria caused over time by free radicals.

Acetyl-L-carnitine and L-carnitine are two slightly different forms of the same molecule, and scientists have used supplements of both of these in human studies. Carnitine is a vitaminlike nutrient found in protein that helps move fats through the mitochondria to where they are burned for energy. Without sufficient carnitine, there is not an adequate transport of fatty acids to the mitochondria. This deficit re - sults in low levels of energy production.

Acetyl-L-Carnitine
A form of the amino acid L-carnitine.

Because of its action in the mitochondria, acetyl-L-carnitine can help to halt the damage to mitochondria and prevent or reverse age-related conditions and changes. Dr. Tory M. Hagen of Oregon State University has conducted major clinical experiments on both acetyl-L-carnitine and the antioxidant alpha-lipoic acid, which also is very active in the mitochondria. He has discovered that tuning up the mitochondria may be a way to delay the onset of age-related problems and may even reverse damage that has already occurred. Acetyl-L-carnitine shows the most promise for heart health, chronic fatigue, and neurological disorders.

A Healthy Heart

Deficiencies of carnitine can lead to serious problems. These include obesity, fatigue, and elevated triglycerides. Long researched for its ability to increase energy in patients with heart disease, acetyl-L-carnitine is associated with higher levels of ATP in portions of the heart muscle when the heart is under stress. In other words, it acts to energize the heart. Furthermore, L-carnitine im proves function of the heart in diabetic animals in which L-carnitine levels are decreased, and in nondiabetic humans who have ischemic heart disease.

There is also evidence that carnitine may be helpful in recovery from open-heart surgery. In a trial conducted on newborn rabbits, which was reported in the *Annals of Thoracic Surgery*, re searchers from the Heart Institute of Japan found that supplementation with carnitine was helpful with fatty acid metabolism after open heart surgery.

In another study, rats that received a diet consisting of fats for fifteen hours, along with an orally administered dose of 500 mg/kg of L-carnitine experienced a decrease in blood triglyceride levels. Triglycerides are compounds that consist of three fatty acids and glycerol. They are the form in which fat is stored in the body and the primary type of fat in the diet. High levels of triglycer-ides are a major risk factor for heart disease and stroke.

Triglycerides *Compounds that consist of three fatty acids and glycerol.*

Relief from Chronic Fatigue Syndrome

Chronic fatigue syndrome is a complicated con-dition characterized by severe, unrelenting fatigue and a variety of other symptoms such as head-aches and impaired memory and concentration. People often suffer for years from this syndrome, which can be debilitating. It severely impacts the quality of life, and sufferers often find it impossi-ble to continue working at a regular job. Many face the frustration of thinking they will never feel well again. Quite a few studies show that there is an association between low levels of L-carnitine and chronic fatigue syndrome.

In a study conducted by the Chronic Fatigue Syndrome Center and Department of Research at Mercy Hospital and Medical Center in Chicago, twelve out of eighteen chronic fatigue patients improved after receiving L-carnitine supplements. The study showed that L-carnitine helped to re-duce physical fatigue as well as to improve mood and mental fatigue.

Another study involved twenty-eight patients with chronic fatigue syndrome who were given either 3 grams of carnitine daily or an antiviral drug for twenty-eight weeks. The men and women who took carnitine showed significant improve-ment according to all measures for improvement, while none of the patients who took the antiviral drug showed improvements.

Benefits for the Brain

Acetyl-L-carnitine also has been found to be beneficial to optimal neurological function. In addition to transporting fats into the mitochondria, acetyl-L-carnitine assists in the production of acetylcholine, which is one of the body's major neurotransmitters.

Neuro-transmitters
Chemical substances that transmit nerve signals between brain cells.

You can think of neurotransmitters like electrical circuits; in order for our brains and bodies to function optimally, the circuit cannot have a break in it—the impulse must make its connection. Because of this neurological function, acetyl-L-carnitine is believed to be highly effective in the treatment of Alzheimer's disease, senility, memory impairment, and nerve damage due to diabetes.

The *Annals of the New York Academy of Science* has noted that acetyl-L-carnitine is considered useful in the treatment of the senile dementia associated with Alzheimer's disease because of its ability to serve as a precursor for the neurotransmitter acetylcholine, as well as because of its ability to support cellular function in the mitochondria. The authors based their hypothesis on studies conducted on animals as well as on observations of a significant decrease of carnitine in the brains of people who died from Alzheimer's disease.

A single-blind clinical trial was conducted on 481 elderly individuals with mild mental impairment to test the effectiveness of acetyl-L-carnitine in the treatment of mental decline in the elderly. The trial involved four phases. In one phase, the subjects were given a placebo for twenty days; in two phases, they were administered 1,500 mg per day of acetyl-L-carnitine for ninety days; and in the last phase, they were given thirty more days of placebo treatment. After each phase, the subjects were given tests to evaluate specific cognitive performances. The results showed a significant increase in cognitive function at the end of treatment with acetyl-L-carnitine as well as improvements in memory and emotions. The researchers concluded that acetyl-L-carnitine may be effective in treating dementia.

Diabetics often suffer from peripheral neuropathy, which is nerve fiber damage and associated sensory loss. Sensory nerves are particularly susceptible to the effects of diabetes. Acetyl-L-carnitine can prevent impairment in peripheral nerves. Researchers have reported that rats treated with the nutrient experienced significant reduction of substance P loss in the sciatic nerves and lumbar spinal cord. Substance P is a neuropeptide, a particular type of brain chemical.

Acetyl-L-Carnitine and Alpha-Lipoic Acid: Stronger in Combination

Perhaps the most significant evidence for the efficacy of acetyl-L-carnitine as an anti-aging supplement has come through a series of experiments that were recently conducted at Oregon State University and at the University of California, Berkeley, and Children's Hospital Oakland Research Institute by Drs. Tory M. Hagen, Bruce N. Ames, and Jiankang Liu. In one study, Dr. Hagen and his colleagues fed groups of young and old laboratory rats either acetyl-L-carnitine or the antioxidant alpha-lipoic acid, or a combination of these nutrients. The nutrients were selected for the study because both acetyl-L-carnitine and alpha-lipoic acid (which will be discussed in Chapter 3) enhance energy production in the mitochondria. The researchers hypothesized that because acetyl-L-carnitine can increase free-radical levels, combining it with a strong antioxidant such as alpha-lipoic acid—one of the few antioxidants that can penetrate mitochondria—would increase beneficial effects. Acetyl-L-carnitine increases free radicals as a byproduct of higher cellular energy production. But again, the researchers believed that lipoic acid would further increase cellular energy levels, but also diminish free radicals.

And that is exactly what happened. After two to four weeks of receiving the supplements, the old rats were rejuvenated. Their physical activity levels doubled, with energy levels approaching those of young rats that did not take any supplements. Even energy levels in young rats receiving the supplement increased by a third. In some cases, the researchers found reversals in memory loss. The effects were strongest for the group of rats given both nutrients, and the researchers compared the results to a seventy-five year old person having the vigor of a forty-five or fifty year old.

In another study, Drs. Ames and Jiankang Liu found that the enzyme carnitine acetyltransferase is less active in old rats and that it binds less tightly to acetyl-L-carnitine. This enzyme is involved in burning fats for energy in the mitochondria and it declines with age. In their experiments, the researchers supplemented the rats' diets with acetyl-L-carnitine or a combination of acetyl-L-carnitine and alpha-lipoic acid.

The results? The treatment restored the enzyme's activity level to close to that of young rats and restored binding to acetyl-L-carnitine. According to Dr. Ames, these studies show that in the combination therapy, the acetyl-L-carnitine protects the protein and boosts the activity of the enzyme carnitine acetyltransferase, while the alpha-lipoic acid destroys oxygen free radicals. It is like taking an enemy on from two fronts.

And in a third study, Drs. Liu, Hagen, Ames,

and colleagues fed old rats a similar diet of the two supplements and then tested their memories. Supplementation improved spatial and temporal memory and lowered oxidative damage in the area of the brain important for memory—the hippocampus. The researchers concluded that tuning up the mitochondria through supplementation with acetyl-L-carnitine and alpha-lipoic acid can delay the onset of age-related problems and may, at times, reverse those changes.

Guidelines for Supplementation

Food sources of L-carnitine include organ meats, fish, and milk products. However, experts recommend taking pharmaceutical grade supplements of amino acid-like substances such as L-carnitine—especially for vegetarians who may be more at risk for deficiencies.

In general, the encapsulated powdered forms are particularly good for easy digestion. L-carnitine should be taken on an empty stomach with some juice. (Taking amino acids with meals will disrupt absorption.) It is also recommended that you not eat for thirty minutes before or after taking an amino acid supplement. For anti-aging benefits, 1 to 3 grams of carnitine daily can help. The acetyl-L form more effectively crosses the blood-brain barrier and, therefore, is more easily assimilated.

CHAPTER 3

ALPHA-LIPOIC ACID

As mentioned in Chapter 2, alpha-lipoic acid is a strong antioxidant that is active in the mitochondria. Its effectiveness as a free-radical scavenger is one of the major reasons it is considered an excellent anti-aging nutrient, especially when combined with acetyl-L-carnitine (see Chapter 2). In addition, alpha-lipoic acid is instrumental in converting glucose to energy and in lowering and stabilizing blood glucose levels. This helps to protect against and treat diabetes, a disease that accelerates the aging process.

Antioxidants
Groups of vitamins, minerals, and enzymes that protect against damage caused by free radicals.

A Powerhouse Antioxidant

Alpha-lipoic acid is a vitaminlike substance with antioxidant properties. Because it is found in all of the body's cells, but is produced in the body in only very small amounts, we must also obtain this nutrient either from our food or from supplements. Foods rich in alpha-lipoic acid include broccoli and meats. Because it is soluble both in water and in fat, alpha-lipoic acid is absorbed easily and can cross cell membranes, making it more powerful than many other antioxidants, which provide protection only outside the cell. Alpha-lipoic acid's ability to cross through cell membranes means that it can attack a greater variety of free radicals in the body. Its tiny size enables it to burrow into the nucleus of a cell and protect against free-radical damage to DNA, which is the cause of many serious chronic diseases, such as cancer.

You can also think of alpha-lipoic acid as a great defender of other antioxidants. For example, it acts to protect glutathione in the body. Glutathione is a compound made from the three amino acids cysteine, glutamic acid, and glycine. Found in the liver, it plays an important role in protecting against radiation and other environmental toxins. In addition, glutathione helps to recycle vitamin C and vitamin E after they have done their work destroying free radicals.

Alpha-lipoic acid's great ability as an antioxidant has made it an effective agent for the treatment or prevention of a number of conditions related to oxidative damage. The antioxidant is effective for combatting AIDS, alcoholism, cancer, and heavy-metal poisoning. Most notably, alpha-lipoic supplementation has been used extensively to treat diabetics for more than two decades in Germany, particularly to treat the nerve and kidney damage related to the disease. While more long-term studies are warranted, this documented long-term use in Europe makes scientists optimistic about alpha-lipoic acid's safety, according to researchers at Harvard.

Glycation

Result of blood sugar reacting spontaneously with proteins to form cross-linking that causes tissue damage.

Effective for Diabetes

Diabetes, which kills an estimated 200,000 people each year, ravages the diabetic's body, causing it to age more rapidly than is normal. This devastation is due primarily to glycation. Besides damaging tissue, this also can result in clogged arteries and kidney problems.

People with diabetes are at greater risk for developing a number of health-threatening and potentially fatal conditions, including heart disease, stroke, and pneumonia. Moreover, 82,000 people each year undergo amputations of legs and feet due to reduced circulation in the lower extremities caused by diabetes. In addition, an estimated 12,000 to 24,000 diabetics will suffer from diabetes-related eye disease and blindness, and 38,000 people will develop kidney failure. The Centers for Disease Control and Prevention predicts that controlling blood pressure and the levels of glucose in the blood would reduce kidney failure in diabetics by 50 percent.

The nutrient alpha-lipoic acid plays a key role in converting glucose to ATP—the cellular form of energy. By helping to transform glucose into energy and increasing the effectiveness of insulin, alpha-lipoic acid helps to combat insulin-resistance and increase insulin sensitivity (the ability of insulin to transport glucose from the blood).

In a recent study conducted at the University of Tuebingen, Germany, seventy-four diabetic patients were given 600 mg of alpha-lipoic acid supplements each day. The patients showed stimulated insulin activity, which lowered and stabilized their glucose levels. Supplementation also increased insulin sensitivity and glucose tolerance.

In another study, researchers at the City Hospital in Baden-Baden, Germany, wanted to see if alpha-lipoic acid, used frequently to treat diabetic nerve pain and damage, would enhance insulin's disposal of glucose. Thirteen patients who were of comparable age and had approximately the same amount of insulin resistance at the beginning of the study received either alpha-lipoic acid or a different substance. The group that received the alpha-lipoic acid experienced a significant increase in the body's ability to use insulin to dispose of glucose. The control group (the group that did not receive alpha-lipoic acid) did not experience any significant result. This was the first clinical study to demonstrate that alpha-lipoic acid increases glucose disposal.

Other Potential Benefits

The degenerative processes we recognize as aging also are associated with reduced levels of glutathione; as mentioned earlier, alpha-lipoic acid helps to protect glutathione levels in the body. Researchers at the University of Madras in India, working on the premise that aging is a failure to maintain a state of balance (homeostasis) under stress, found that when aged rats were given alpha-lipoic acid, they experienced a reduction in free radicals and an increase in the activity and level of the glutathione system.

Homeostasis
The tendency of the physiological system to maintain internal stability.

A recent issue of *Harvard Women's Heath Watch* reported that studies conducted on rodents have indicated that alpha-lipoic acid prevented hearing loss and reduced brain damage after stroke. Supplementation with alpha-lipoic acid also improved the memory and cognitive functions of older mice. Clinical trials are currently underway on humans to determine if the supplement can improve not only short-term memory and cognition, but also muscle strength and metabolism as we age.

Last, a study conducted at Canada's University of Western Ontario looked at the effect of a number of antioxidants and cysteine-elevating drugs on the eye lens damage following exposure to radiation levels that approximated those levels astronauts, jet crews, and military personnel might encounter. Alpha-lipoic acid was found to protect the study's participants against radiation-associated protein damage. The study's researchers concluded that it was possible that antioxidants can provide protection against cataracts.

Dosage Recommendation

In general, 50 mg of alpha-lipoic acid daily will provide excellent antioxidant support. People with insulin resistance or Syndrome X may benefit from 200 mg daily. In Europe, physicians commonly prescribe 600 mg daily to treat diabetic nerve disease. Although these dosages of alpha-lipoic acid are safe, they may reduce requirements for drugs that lower blood sugar. If you take such medications, please work with your physician to adjust the dosage.

CHAPTER 4

MELATONIN

Hormones, which are released by the endocrine system, regulate so many of the body's functions. To name a few of these functions, they affect the reproductive system, sex drive, growth, and moods. Melatonin is a hormone that is made by the neurotransmitter serotonin and secreted by the pineal gland. Its primary function is synchronizing the timing for the secretion of other hormones.

Your body releases hormones according to a circadian rhythm, which is the natural twenty-four-hour cycle for biological processes. You can think of your body's release of hormones as being set by an inner body clock. At various specific times each day, your body releases particular hormones to receptive organs or tissues.

Hormone
A compound secreted by the endocrine glands that affects the functions of particular receptive organs or tissues.

In addition to overseeing the timing of hormone secretions, melatonin affects how awake or asleep you feel. In fact, it is often referred to as the great sleep hormone: its efficacy as a sleeping aid and for jet lag relief has been well documented.

Melatonin is also a strong antioxidant that has the ability to permeate any cell in the body, providing special protection of the nucleus (the central part of your cells, which contains your genetic materials) against free radicals. It also is able to stimulate the transport of electrons and the production of ATP in the mitochondria.

The rhythms of melatonin production are set by light. Levels of melatonin increase during the dark of night and decrease in daylight. It is one of the substances that your body produces in great quantity while you are young, but which declines significantly as you age. In fact, levels of melatonin begin to drop as early as puberty.

Connection to Human Growth Hormone

As an anti-aging supplement, melatonin may be particularly effective because of its connection to human growth hormone, which also declines once puberty hits. Higher levels of human growth hormone are associated with youth and vitality. Some researchers believe that by increasing melatonin levels, your body is stimulated to release more human growth hormone. But this remains unproved. However, melatonin may promote longevity: studies in rats have shown that their life span increased from twenty-five months to thirty-one months when given supplements of melatonin.

There is evidence that melatonin supplements can be effective in improving cognitive function, preventing and treating neurological diseases such as Alzheimer's disease, improving sleeping ability, and improving heart health.

Improves Cognitive Ability

Scientists believe that melatonin is particularly promising in combating damage done to brain tissue because the hormone is rapidly taken up by the brain. Melatonin has been shown to be effective in scavenging a very toxic radical known as hydroxyl radical and is more efficient than vitamin E in neutralizing the peroxyl radical, another toxic brain radical.

Parkinson's disease and Alzheimer's disease result at least in part from the oxidative stress caused by free radicals in your brain. The brain is particularly vulnerable to free-radical attack. In its enormous use of oxygen, it is the organ that generates the greatest number of free radicals. In order to understand the way melatonin acts to protect the brain, researchers from the Max-Planck-Institute of Psychiatry in Munich, Germany, compared the ability of melatonin and its precursor, normelatonin (a form of serotonin), to protect brain cells against oxidative stress. They discovered that both melatonin and normelatonin protected against neurodegenerative disorders such as Alzheimer's disease and Parkinson's disease.

In addition, patients with dementia often show an absence of melatonin, and Alzheimer's patients show diminished functioning of the pineal gland. After being administered supplementation with melatonin, older people experienced a significant decrease in confusion and agitation during the evening hours. In addition, aged people with sleep disorders were better able to remember things after being given melatonin. In a case report of identical twins with Alzheimer's disease, melatonin administration had a beneficial effect on the course of the disease.

Help for the Sleep Deprived

Tossing and turning at night, longing for sleep that refuses to come, cursing the clock by your bed as the numbers move toward morning: Anyone who has had difficulty sleeping knows how disruptive and detrimental it is to your sense of well-being, energy levels, and emotional state. Getting enough sleep is essential to our health, and there is an association between lack of sleep and illness, even death. In fact, older people with sleep disorders have 1.6 to 2 times higher mortality rates than those who sleep well.

Many of us may think of a good night's sleep as a luxury. Our lives can be so overscheduled and we're always finding ways to squeeze more into the set twenty-four hours that constitute a day. Often, we shave off the minutes and hours that we will allow ourselves for rest. But sleep is critical if we are to push back the aging process. It rejuvenates the body (it is during sleep that human growth hormone, which stimulates muscle growth and helps to maintain a lean body composition, is released) and is essential for physical and mental vitality.

Yet, not only does sleep affect how we age, but also aging affects the way we sleep, more than any other factor, including illness and depression. When we age, there are several changes to our circadian rhythms. Major changes occur to our sleep-wake cycle, resulting in older people's being awake more during the night and sleeping more during the day. Nearly 30 percent of all people over age fifty report sleeping problems.

Circadian Rhythm

A person's natural biological rhythm over twenty-four hours, which influences the normal secretion of hormones.

Not only does the quantity of our sleep decline with age, but the quality does, as well. Aging also leads to increased awakenings during the night—with difficulty falling back to sleep—and early awakening in the morning. The increase in the number of awakenings during the night provokes a decrease in the amount and duration of REM (rapid eye movement) sleep, the deep restorative sleep that enables us to awake feeling fresh and invigorated.

Melatonin can help you to get the good sleep that you need to feel and look young at any age. The secretion of melatonin in your body, with its nocturnal peaks and daytime lows, regulates your sleep cycles. When working well at the appropriate levels, it causes you to feel sleepy during the night and awake during the day. For this reason, the insomnia in older people may be caused at least in part by the diminished levels of melatonin. Studies have shown that supplementation with melatonin can help to improve sleep, with a low probability of undesirable side effects.

A variety of dosages and preparations of melatonin have been used in experiments to stimulate sleep in older people. Researchers at Massachusetts Institute of Technology studied a group of adults over the age of fifty. Half of those studied had insomnia; the rest said they slept normally. The purpose of the study was to determine if oral doses of melatonin could restore blood levels of melatonin and increase sleep.

The study involved administering in random order, a placebo and three dosage levels of melatonin (0.1, 0.3, and 3.0 mg) orally one half hour before bedtime for seven consecutive nights. The trial was double blind (meaning that neither the researchers nor the people studied knew who were actually getting melatonin supplements or who were getting a placebo until the results were analyzed).

The outcome of the clinical trial, which was reported in the *Journal of Clinical Endocrinology and Metabolism,* indicated that all three dosages of melatonin improved sleep; however, while the 0.3 mg dose restored blood plasma melatonin levels to normal, the higher dose of 3.0 mg raised levels too much, disturbing the circadian rhythm of melatonin levels so that they remained high even during daylight. For melatonin to function as it should, its levels should decrease during the day. Based on these results, the researchers recommended using the lowest effective dose of a hormone to treat deficiencies with the goal being to raise levels to normal.

In fact, now several studies have found that administering melatonin in oral dosages of as little as 0.3 mg is sufficient to promote and sustain sleep in insomniacs. In another study, melatonin administered in a timed-release formula also showed promise in improving sleep among insomniacs who were deficient in this nutrient.

Cardiovascular Benefits

As the human body ages, its susceptibility to heart disease increases. A summary of research over the last ten years, reviewed by scientists at the Institute of Endocrinology, Medical University of Lodz in Poland, indicates that melatonin plays a role in heart health. Vascular receptors to which melatonin binds were identified, and shown to be linked with melatonin's ability to constrict or dilate blood vessels. Research also has shown that patients with heart disease, in particular those with higher risk of heart attack and sudden death, produce melatonin in low rates. Research on rats also showed that melatonin protects the heart after ischemia, a restriction of blood flow.

Melatonin also may be effective at lowering cholesterol levels. As we age, our cholesterol levels often increase, with levels of LDL cholesterol (the low-density, artery-clogging kind) rising and levels of HDL cholesterol (the high-density, cleansing form of cholesterol) falling. Ideally, your LDL cholesterol levels should be under 100 and your HDL levels should be greater than 35. Reports indicate that people with high levels of LDL have low levels of melatonin, and that melatonin can prevent formation of cholesterol by 38 percent and reduce LDL levels by 42 percent.

Along with elevated cholesterol levels, high blood pressure or hypertension (typically defined as greater than 140/90) puts you at greater risk for heart disease and stroke. Research shows that administering melatonin in 1-mg doses can lower blood pressure to the normal range. Explanations for melatonin's ability to lower blood pressure include its direct effect on the brain, its antioxidant properties, and its ability to relax muscle in the aorta.

Dosage Recommendations

As supplemental hormones go, melatonin is probably the safest, and it is available in the United States without a prescription. However, it still should be used carefully to minimize side effects.

Take melatonin about one hour or so before bedtime in order to correspond with the natural rise in melatonin in the evening. Although 3 mg is often recommended, this is probably too high a dosage for most people, and it is certainly greater than the levels that naturally occur in most people. Too much melatonin might negatively affect your body's circadian rhythms, and large doses can cause grogginess and drowsiness the following day. For this reason, limit your supplementation to 0.1 mg to 0.3 mg (or one-tenth to one-third milligram). Of course, if your physician prescribes a higher dosage, follow his or her instructions.

In addition to supplementation, you can also try to maintain your melatonin levels by eating regular meals, eating lightly at night, avoiding stimulants like caffeine, and avoiding vigorous exercise close to your bedtime.

CHAPTER 5

B-COMPLEX VITAMINS

Without vitamins, our bodies would not be able to function. In short, we could not live. These micronutrients assist in a spectrum of biochemical processes—from synthesizing macronutrients for energy to protecting the circulatory system. Although we know that we need vitamins (mothers have been telling their children to make sure they take their daily vitamin from day one, right?), we still feel unsure about how much of a particular vitamin is the right dosage: Is the recommended dietary allowance (RDA) adequate?

That's a tricky question, because the RDA assumes that most of our vitamins will come from food intake. While it is *desirable* to obtain most of our nutrients directly from the foods we eat, as a practical matter, it is not always possible to get adequate amounts this way. This is especially true as we age and our ability to absorb nutrients diminishes. Also, the RDA levels are good to prevent deficiencies of a particular vitamin, but do not take into account that higher doses may be warranted today to help the body counteract the increase in environmental toxins, the stress of modern life, and the increase in consumption of mass-produced processed foods that can have reduced nutritional value. It's easy

Vitamin
A compound, essential to health, that helps to release energy from food and acts as a catalyst for many metabolic functions.

to see why it may be prudent to take vitamin supplements.

We can think of the B-complex vitamins as a powerhouse team, with each player contributing its own talents to enhance your well-being and get you into the winners circle of good health. B-complex vitamins perform a variety of important metabolic functions that include maintaining blood sugar levels; the health of your hair, skin, eyes, and circulatory system; and brain function. Many of the B vitamins also are involved in energy production, helping to convert fats, proteins, and carbohydrates into energy.

There are two general groups of vitamins; those that are fat-soluble and those that are water-soluble. Fat-soluble vitamins (A, D, E, and K) can be stored for long periods of time in the body's fatty tissue and liver. The B-complex vitamins, as well as vitamin C, are water-soluble, which means that they are excreted within a few days; they cannot be stored. Therefore, the water-soluble vitamins must be replaced often, preferably daily. In addition, your ability to absorb B vitamins decreases as you age, making it even more important to ensure you have adequate intake of the B vitamins.

Getting to Know the B Team

The B-complex group includes vitamin B_1 (thiamine), vitamin B_2 (riboflavin), vitamin B_3 (niacin, niacinamide, nicotinic acid), vitamin B_5 (panto - thenic acid), vitamin B_6 (pyridoxine), and vitamin B_{12} (cyanocobalamin). Each B vitamin plays an important role in supporting your metabolic health.

Vitamin B_1

Vitamin B_1 helps maintain circulatory health, proper digestion, muscle tone, and optimal brain function and metabolizes carbohydrates.

It is found in foods such as brown rice, pea-nuts, whole grains, and legumes.

Vitamin B₂

Vitamin B_2 helps your body produce antibodies, is instrumental in cell repair, forms red blood cells, and prevents cataracts. It also helps to provide oxygen in a variety of tissues, including your hair, nails, and skin.

Sources of vitamin B_2 include cheese, egg yolks, poultry, and spinach.

Vitamin B₃

Vitamin B_3 is essential for healthy skin and circulation. It also helps to metabolize nutrients, helps lower blood cholesterol and triglyceride levels, produces hydrochloric acid for proper digestion, and can enhance cognitive function.

Foods rich in vitamin B_3 (specifically niacin) include beef liver, broccoli, fish, poultry, peanuts, and wheat germ.

Vitamin B₅

Vitamin B_5 is called the antistress vitamin. It assists in protein and red blood cell formation, helps in the production of the adrenal hormones and antibodies, and helps to convert nutrients into energy.

It is found in meat, poultry, fish, whole grains, and legumes.

Vitamin B₆

Vitamin B_6 is vital for both physical and mental health. Some of its important functions include aiding in the production of red blood cells, facilitating normal brain function, and synthesizing RNA and DNA. It also activates many enzymes and helps the body absorb vitamin B_{12}. Finally, and perhaps most important when it comes to anti-aging, vitamin B_6 inhibits the production of homocysteine, a toxic substance that leads to heart disease (this is discussed in greater detail below).

Food sources include poultry, fish, organ meats, nuts, legumes, and whole grains.

Vitamin B_{12}

Vitamin B_{12} prevents anemia and nerve damage. It also aids in digestion and the synthesis of proteins. It also is associated with the production of the neurotransmitter acetylcholine. In addition, vitamin B_{12} is used in the production of DNA and RNA. It is common for older people to have trouble absorbing vitamin B_{12}, which can lead to a deficiency.

This vitamin is obtained primarily from animal sources, such as kidney, liver, poultry, eggs, milk, and seafood.

B Vitamins to Reduce Homocysteine for Cardiovascular Health

Homocysteine is an amino acid produced naturally by the body. Normally, homocysteine is then changed into other amino acids for use in the body. If it is not, and its levels remain too high (above 12 µmol per L), it can irritate blood vessels and lead to atherosclerosis (blocked arteries).

Homocysteine
A toxic amino acid, which can increase the risk of blood vessel blockage and contribute to the deposit of cholesterol around the heart.

It is estimated that 20 percent of people with heart disease have high levels of homocysteine. Therefore, your homocysteine levels are an indicator of how much at risk you are for developing heart disease. Levels of homocysteine can be tested through a simple blood test and doctors are now increasingly making such a test part of their routine blood workup.

Reducing the levels of homocysteine in your body can decrease your risk of heart disease.

If you have a close relative who has developed heart disease at a younger than expected age, you are at increased risk for developing the disease yourself. Tracking your homocysteine levels may help decrease your risk. One study, conducted at National Hospital in Norway, found that children (aged eight to twelve) whose father, grandfather, or uncle died of premature cardiovascular disease had higher levels of cholesterol and homocysteine. Based on these results, the researchers recommended modifying levels of homocysteine in the diet of younger people who have a family history of heart disease.

It is common for people who undergo angioplasty, a procedure in which blocked blood vessels are unclogged with a catheter, to have to have the procedure repeated down the road because of a return of the blockage. The *New England Journal of Medicine* reported that patients treated with a combination of folic acid, vitamin B_6, and vitamin B_{12} benefitted from reduced homocysteine levels and a lower incidence of subsequent cardiovascular problems. The treatment with vitamins also was recommended for patients undergoing angioplasty.

While it has not been scientifically proven that high levels of homocysteine actually cause cardiovascular disease, scientific studies have demonstrated a definite association between high levels and increased risk of heart disease as well as other illnesses. *Stroke* reported the results of a study conducted in Northern Ireland in which researchers compared levels of homocysteine in groups of people who had suffered a stroke, had vascular dementia, or had Alzheimer's disease with a control group. The researchers discovered that all three disease groups had higher levels of

plasma homocysteine than those without any of
the diseases.

B Vitamins to Protect against Dementia

High levels of homocysteine have been associated not only with cardiovascular health, but also
with deterioration of mental capacity. The *New
England Journal of Medicine* recently reported
the results of a study of 1,092 older men and
women (the average age was seventy-six) who
did not suffer from dementia at the beginning of
the study. After eight years, dementia developed
in 111 of the people, 83 of whom were broadly
diagnosed with Alzheimer's disease. (It should be
noted that a conclusive diagnosis of Alzheimer's
disease is possible only via autopsy. In this study,
five subjects received a clinical diagnosis of Alzheimer's disease confirmed at autopsy; 67 subjects were diagnosed with "probably Alzheimer's";
and 11 with "possible Alzheimer's.") Those who
developed dementia were more likely to have increased levels of homocysteine than those who
did not develop the disease.

Research suggests that deficiencies in the B
vitamins are common, particularly in older adults.
People who have deficiencies of vitamin B are
more apt to have increased levels of homocysteine because vitamins B_6 and B_{12} help the body
process homocysteine. There is also evidence
that supplementation with B vitamins can offer
protection by lowering plasma levels of homocysteine.

It is estimated that Alzheimer's disease afflicts
6 to 8 percent of all people over age sixty-five
and it accounts for more than 50 percent of the
cases of dementia in older people. The preva-
lence of the disease is on the rise. Many studies
have indicated that free radicals play a role in the

genesis of this disease by causing accelerated damage to cells of the nervous system.

A major article, published in the *American Journal of Clinical Nutrition,* reviewed several recent studies to determine the relationship between Alzheimer's disease and possible protective effects of nutritional factors—in particular, folate, vitamin B_{12}, and vitamin B_6. The authors of the article noted that research has shown a relationship between cognitive ability and blood levels of B vitamins; and that people with Alzheimer's disease commonly have low vitamin B_{12} levels. It is possible that B vitamin and folate deficiency may interfere with the metabolism of neurotransmitters, thereby negatively affecting brain metabolism and causing cognitive problems.

The authors also referenced the homocysteine factor: in particular, that high levels of the amino acid have been linked to increased risk for both cardiovascular and brain diseases. It is thought that the damage to blood vessel walls caused by excess homocysteine may, in part, be responsible for damage to cognitive function as well (it is known that cerebrovascular tears can cause neurologic disorders). Based on these observations, and on the results of studies of homocysteine concentrations in people with and without dementia, the authors concluded that B-vitamin supplementation may provide protection against Alzheimer's disease, and that more clinical trials were desirable.

Vitamin B to Boost Cognitive Function

As you age, vitamin B also may help to improve your brain power in general—your memory and concentration. One study conducted by the Human Nutrition Research Center on Aging at Tufts University in Boston looked at seventy men, aged fifty-four to eighty-one and the relationship between their blood levels of homocysteine and vitamins B_{12}, B_6, and folate and their scores on a group of cognitive tests. The study found that those with higher concentrations of vitamin B_6 performed better in tests of memory.

The *Journal of the American Medical Association (JAMA)* reported the results of another trial that evaluated the link between cognitive ability and nutrition in a group of 260 independent men and women over age sixty. The group was given the Halstead-Reitan Categories Test, which evaluates abstract thinking ability, and the Wechsler Memory Test. Researchers found that those people with low levels of vitamins C or B_{12} did not perform as well on both tests. In addition, those with low levels of folic acid scored worse on the abstract thinking test.

Dosage Recommendations

The B vitamins should be taken together in a single capsule form, but you can also take more of a particular B vitamin if you have a specific problem you need to address. A B-complex supplement that includes more than the RDA of each vitamin is recommended. Be sure to read labels carefully so that you know you are purchasing vitamins that are derived from natural sources, which are more easily absorbed and assimilated.

CHAPTER 6

CALCIUM

Calcium is an essential mineral for building bones and teeth and for maintaining their strength. It also is important for proper muscle contraction, transmission of nerve impulses, blood clotting, and the maintenance of cell membranes. We have more calcium in our bodies than any other mineral. Calcium helps us to look and feel young. Among the many symptoms of calcium deficiency are aching joints, brittle nails, a pasty complexion, and decaying teeth.

As we age, and our bone tissue is dissolved and replaced, we lose calcium. Menopausal women in particular need more calcium to offset the loss of estrogen, which is a hormone that protects bone density by helping to promote the deposit of calcium in bone. The Recommended Dietary Allowance of calcium for adults is 1,000 mg for men and women age nineteen to fifty, and 1,200 mg for those over age fifty. Scientists from the Centers for Disease Control estimate that adults over age sixty are severely deficient in calcium—nearly two-thirds have daily intakes below the recommended doses. In addition, a recent review of the available science by the American Academy of Pediatrics asserted that children and adolescents are not getting enough calcium; the group supported recommendations that preteens and adolescents have calcium levels of 1,200–1,500 mg per day.

With regard to the RDA, one consideration should be kept in mind: the amount of calcium you need depends upon how much of it your body actually absorbs into your bloodstream and tissues. If you take more than you can absorb, you are not doing yourself any good, as explained below. Your body's ability to absorb calcium will vary depending on your age, any health conditions you may have, and your diet (vitamin D helps your body absorb calcium). Check with your healthcare provider to determine the appropriate amount of calcium for your body.

The Proper Amount Is Essential

When it comes to calcium supplementation, a delicate balance must be struck. It is essential that you get the appropriate amounts of calcium: the right amount can offer you protection, but too much can actually leave you more vulnerable to diseases such as arthritis and heart disease. This is because excess calcium is not simply excreted by the body the way that your body may excrete excess amounts of certain vitamins, such as vitamin C. Instead, excess calcium may gather in the arteries, potentially causing them to clog, or it may collect in your joints and lead to arthritis, or in the kidney and leave you at more risk for kidney stones.

Minerals
Naturally occurring substances that enable the performance of vital bodily functions, includ - ing building bones and connective tissues.

In fact, in order to prevent the collection of excess calcium in the arteries, drugs known as calcium-channel blockers are sometimes used. There have been reports however, that calcium-channel blockers may be harmful to people with diabetes or high blood pressure. As an alternative to these pharmaceuticals, it may be possible for you to take magnesium, which also can block calcium accumulation and help regulate heart rate. Talk to your doctor to determine whether magnesium supplementation may be right for you.

To prevent blockage caused by calcium, be wise about your intake of this necessary and powerful mineral. A dose of about 500 mg per day of calcium seems to be what the body can absorb best. Remember that too much calcium may be harmful, but the right amounts have protective effects. You just need to strike the right balance.

Osteoporosis

Translated as "porous bone," osteoporosis is a condition characterized by a loss in bone density and bone strength. It is a very serious disease. People with osteoporosis are at great risk for serious injury from falls. The bones of a person with osteoporosis can become so brittle and weak that they cannot withstand even the normal stresses of daily life. The disease has nearly become an epidemic, afflicting 25 million Americans—nearly 10 percent of our population. Close to 80 percent of these are postmenopausal women; close to 20 percent are older men. But this disease has been diagnosed in younger men and women, as well.

Risk factors for osteoporosis include alcohol abuse, recent loss of height (one inch or more), being on your feet for less than three hours a day, cessation of menstrual periods for six months or more (unless you are menopausal), fractures of the wrist (which often are the first signs of osteoporosis), unexplained tooth loss, and a decrease in sex drive. A doctor can diagnosis osteoporosis thorough a bone-mineral density test.

Undoubtedly, you have heard much about calcium—in particular for its potential to prevent osteoporosis. Because calcium is so essential for bone health, many people think that they should take calcium in large amounts to prevent bone loss. This, however is controversial with some studies showing a protective effect and others not. There is some evidence that levels of 500 mg per day is optimal for good absorption and may help protect your bones.

Calcium may also protect against fractures in women without osteoporosis. *The Journal of Rheumatology* reported the results of a study conducted at Virginia Commonwealth University that compared the development of vertebral fractures in four groups of women: thirty year olds with normal bone density, fifty year olds with borderline osteoporosis, sixty year olds with moderate osteoporosis, and seventy year olds with severe osteoporosis. After ten years of supplementation with calcium and vitamin D, fracture rates in all groups decreased by 30 to 50 percent.

While calcium by itself will not prevent or cure osteoporosis, the National Osteoporosis Foundation recommends it as part of an overall prevention or treatment approach—one that also includes weight-bearing exercise, such as strength training, in order to maintain or increase bone density.

Weight Control and Cancer Prevention

If you are battling to keep your weight under control, here's some interesting news. Recent studies show promise for calcium's ability both to help you control your weight and to protect you against certain cancers. The *Journal of the American College of Nutrition* cited studies that showed that people who consumed less calcium were more overweight and gained more weight during middle age than those who had higher intakes of calcium.

Additional research from the University of Tennessee suggests that when you reduce your caloric intake but have higher levels of calcium, you are more apt to burn fat. The reason for this is that calcium may suppress levels of the substance 1.25-dihydroxyvitamin D, which stimulates fat production in the body. In the October 2001 issue of the *Journal of the American College of Nutrition,* Michael B. Zemel, Ph.D., noted that while there have not been enough large-scale clinical trials on the subject, there is evidence that increasing dietary calcium may result in reduced fat.

Several recent studies also show a link between calcium intake and a lower risk for certain cancers. The Nurses' Health Study showed that calcium in the diet does not affect the risk of breast cancer in women after menopause, but that premenopausal women with higher calcium levels reduced their breast cancer risk by 30 percent when compared with women whose diets contained low levels of calcium.

Calcium appears to be particularly effective in the protection against colon cancer. Colon cancer is a common form of cancer and the second leading cause of all cancer deaths. Possible risk factors for colon cancer include obesity, lack of activity, low fruit and vegetable consumption, alcohol consumption, and cigarette smoking. The risk of developing colon cancer increases as you age, particularly after age fifty. There are several good screening tests available for colon cancer, including colonoscopy and fecal occult blood test, which can help detect colon cancer in its earliest, highly curable stages. If you are over age fifty, speak to your doctor about screening for colon cancer.

In general, you can reduce your risk for this type of cancer by eating a diet that is rich in fruits and vegetables, and which is low in animal fat, calories, and alcohol. While diets high in fiber and vegetables were once touted as being the first line of defense against this disease, some controversy now exists because several well-designed trials did not show a link between reduced colon cancer risk and consumption of vegetables and fiber. However, the evidence for calcium's effectiveness in this area is growing.

The *Journal of the National Cancer Institute* reported that people who consumed higher levels of calcium had a 35 percent less likely chance of developing colon cancer than those with low levels of calcium. Another study that tested the effects of administering 900 mg per day of calcium to forty people at risk for colon cancer also had positive results. Increased dietary calcium, given either as supplements or in the diet in low-fat dairy foods, lowered risk of changes to the colon that can be precursors to colon cancer. Calcium supplements helped to reduce the recurrence of polyps in the colon, which also increases risk for colon cancer.

The *Journal of the American Medical Association* (JAMA) reported the results of a clinical controlled study, conducted by the Department of Medicine, St. Luke's Roosevelt Hospital Center and Columbia University on whether increasing calcium intake alters precancerous changes in the colon. In the randomized controlled study, led by Dr. Peter R. Holt, seventy people who had had a history of polyps in their colon were given low-fat dairy products containing up to 1,200 mg per day of calcium. After six and twelve months of treatment, several indicators of increased risk for colon

Randomized Controlled Study
A scientific study in which members are assigned randomly, and with equal chance, to either a control group or a treatment group in order to prove the effectiveness of a treatment.

cancer were reduced. The researchers concluded that increasing daily intake of calcium in low-fat dairy food reduced risk for precancerous changes to the colon in people with a history of polyps.

They stressed that it was the increased calcium obtained in the low-fat dairy foods that led to the study's positive results, rather than the fact that the diets were simply low in fat. The researchers also noted that this study built on previous research conducted on both rats and humans, which showed that increasing dietary calcium reduces the spread of precancerous colon cells. Obtaining calcium through low-fat sources is important since many of the natural sources of calcium—such as whole milk and cheese—are high in fat and eating such high-fat foods could increase the risk of colon cancer.

Some experts have disagreed with these results, noting that it has not been adequately proved that the calcium per se is responsible for any protective effects. They caution that increasing calcium intake to high levels has been associated with an increased risk of prostate cancer in men. However, this link has not been shown in all studies and there is the possibility that the association found has more to do with consuming too many calories than too much calcium.

Dosage Recommendations

Food sources of calcium include dairy products, European sparkling mineral waters, and leafy green vegetables. Many foods, such as orange juice and cereals, are fortified with calcium. Re - member not to take too much calcium. Supplements of 1,000 mg may be too much, especially if you are getting calcium through your food intake. Instead, doses of no higher than 500 mg may be more appropriate. Also, it may be better to take calcium in small doses throughout the day and before going to sleep at night, rather than in one large daily dose.

Partner with Magnesium

One important note: calcium is a mineral that works in conjunction with magnesium. Magnesium helps your heart muscles to relax, whereas calcium helps your muscles to contract. Both functions are necessary, and there must be a balance between magnesium and calcium in your body. Many people are deficient in magnesium. Consider adding 400 mg of magnesium to your calcium supplement.

CHAPTER 7

COENZYME Q_{10}

There is a lot of good anti-aging news about coenzyme Q_{10} (CoQ_{10}). This coenzyme (also known as ubiquinone) is a potent antioxidant found in the mitochondria of our muscles and organs, particularly in the heart, liver, kidneys, and pancreas. This coenzyme is made or synthesized by the body. In addition, it can be obtained through food sources that include animal meats and seafood.

CoQ_{10} acts as an antioxidant that helps to reduce age-related damage caused by free radicals. Perhaps even more important, it helps the body produce cellular energy in the form of adenosine triphosphate (ATP). CoQ_{10} manufactures cellular energy by shuttling protons and electrons—which contain energy—in the mito-chondria. Its energy-producing function is so im-portant that this powerful coenzyme has been compared to the spark plug of a car—our bodies need CoQ_{10} to ignite our system, to get it going. However, as is the case with many nutrients, the levels of CoQ_{10} in the body decrease as we age.

Anti-Aging Role

Because of its powerful double function as an antioxidant and major energy producer, CoQ_{10} has been the subject of several scientific studies on a wide range of conditions. These studies have shown CoQ_{10} to be quite promising in a number of health-related areas, including improved appearance.

CoQ$_{10}$'s strength as an antioxidant has led to claims that it can prevent damage to the body's collagen and elastin production process. As you age, your body produces less of these connective tissues, which are essential for your skin to have a young, bright, wrinkle-free, full appearance. This is why some people concerned with a youthful appearance may endure collagen injections as they age. That process involves injecting collagen derived from the connective tissue of cows or pigs under the skin in order to temporarily erase wrinkles and plump up the skin. However, such injections are costly, the results temporary, and the process also comes with potential side effects, including allergic reactions, infections, scarring, and partial blindness. CoQ$_{10}$ may produce effects similar to collagen injections, without the adverse reactions. Because CoQ$_{10}$ can protect your collagen and elastin production, it is contained in several health and beauty creams.

Coenzymes
Molecules that help enzymes speed up chemical reactions needed for our bodies to function. They work with enzymes to either join molecules or to separate them.

In addition to the potential cosmetic benefits of CoQ$_{10}$ supplementation, the substance has been widely studied for its healing and protective properties against several age-related illnesses and conditions. These include neurological disease, cancer, and most particularly heart disease and hypertension.

Promise for Neurological Disease

Parkinson's disease is a degenerative neurological disease that usually strikes individuals over age fifty. It may begin with symptoms that are subtle and not very specific—a slight tremor, a general sense of malaise, stiffness in the legs, and balance problems. The disease afflicts more than 50,000 people each year in the United States alone. There is no cure for Parkinson's disease; its course usually runs from between ten to fifteen years, with symptoms progressively worsening.

Researchers at the University of California, San Diego, sought to determine a safe range of doses of CoQ_{10}, and to learn whether the coenzyme could slow down the physical decline of individuals with Parkinson's disease. To test their theory, the investigators gathered eighty people from movement disorders clinics who were in the early stages of Parkinson's disease but who did not yet require any treatment. The patients were randomly assigned to receive either a placebo (sugar pill) or CoQ_{10} treatment in doses of 300, 600, or 1,200 mg per day. The study's participants were evaluated with the Unified Parkinson Disease Rating Scale at the beginning of the study and then again at several intervals over four months.

When the results were analyzed, researchers discovered that patients who received the CoQ_{10} treatment developed less disability than those who received the placebo. While the progress of Parkinson's disease slowed at all three doses of CoQ_{10}, the patients who were assigned the highest dose of 1,200 mg showed the greatest slowing of symptoms or improvement.

In addition, the CoQ_{10} treatment was found to be safe and well tolerated at all three dosages. Based on these results, the study's authors concluded that although a larger study was needed for confirmation, CoQ_{10} shows promise in slowing the progressive deterioration in Parkinson's disease.

Cancer Management

Most of the studies performed on animals have

indicated that CoQ_{10} can enhance the immune system and protect against cancer. These results show some promise for use of this coenzyme in cancer management. Experts note that more human studies on CoQ_{10} in this area are needed before any major conclusions can be drawn. However, there is compelling evidence to indicate that CoQ_{10} can prevent or treat cancer.

The *Harvard Women's Health Letter* notes that patients with certain types of cancer, including cancer of the breast, have lower levels of CoQ_{10} in their bodies than people without the disease. This finding may indicate that CoQ_{10} has a protective effect against breast cancer. It also has been reported that breast cancer patients taking CoQ_{10} along with other antioxidants and fatty acids experienced a partial regression of their tumors.

In one study, reported in *Molecular Aspects of Medicine*, thirty-two high-risk breast cancer patients, aged thirty-two to eighty-one, were given treatment with vitamin C, vitamin E, beta-carotene, selenium, essential fatty acids, and CoQ_{10}. The patients were considered particularly high risk because their tumors had spread to the lymph nodes. The supplemental nutritional treatment was in addition to surgical and standard therapeutic treatment for breast cancer.

The researchers discovered that after eighteen months of treatment, none of the patients died, which was unexpected. In addition, none showed further spread of cancer, and quality of life improved, with no weight loss and less use of painkillers. Six patients even went into partial remission. One of those six received increased amounts of CoQ_{10} (390 mg, compared to 90 mg for the rest). For that patient, the tumor disappeared after one month of additional treatment.

In another case, a woman with breast cancer

underwent nonradical surgery followed by treatment with 300 mg of CoQ_{10}. Three months later, the tumor was no longer detectable and the patient was in excellent condition. Such results support the theory that the bioenergetic activity of CoQ_{10} may help shrink tumors.

Blood Pressure Control

CoQ_{10} is abundant in heart muscle. By far, the greatest evidence of CoQ_{10}'s anti-aging prowess is in the areas of hypertension and heart disease. Well-conducted studies show that CoQ_{10} can help lower high blood pressure and can improve the health of people with cardiovascular diseases, including hypertension, angina, and heart failure.

Hypertension is defined as blood pressure that is 140/90 or higher; ideally, you want your blood pressure to be no higher than 120/80. The first number refers to the systolic phase of your heart muscle's work. This is when your heart muscle contracts in order to push blood through your body. The second number is the diastolic phase, which is when your heart muscle is at rest.

If you have high blood pressure, you are at a much-increased risk for cardiovascular disease, congestive heart failure, and stroke. High blood pressure can be caused by a variety of factors including blocked arteries, high levels of salt or sugar, obesity, and stress. This disease affects more than 50 million adults. It is usually treated with pharmaceuticals such as diuretics or beta-blockers, which help to lower pressure but which can also cause side effects such as fatigue and headaches.

Congestive Heart Failure

Congestive heart failure is the inability of the heart to effectively pump blood through the body. It most often results from a heart attack (myocardial infarction) or long-term high blood pressure.

Several studies have shown that CoQ_{10} can lower the blood pressure of people with hypertension. Scientists believe that CoQ_{10} works by fixing an abnormality in your body's metabolic process, which in turn causes blood pressure to drop. For example, it may lower cholesterol levels, which can also have the effect of lowering blood pressure.

In one study, ten patients with high blood pressure experienced drops in both systolic and diastolic pressure after taking 100 mg of CoQ_{10} each day over a ten-week period. In addition, their cholesterol levels fell and their arteries were more open, allowing blood to flow more freely.

Scientists at the Department of Veterans Affairs Medical Center, Boise, Idaho, investigated the effectiveness of oral supplements of CoQ_{10} in lowering blood pressure. The study's researchers worked with a group of forty-six men and thirty-seven women who had systolic hypertension. In a twelve-week, randomized, double-blind controlled trial, they administered two 60-mg doses a day of CoQ_{10} to half of the group, while the other half received a placebo. At the end of the study, those who received the CoQ_{10} had reduced their blood pressure by a mean of 17.8 mm Hg. Because of these positive results, the authors of the study concluded that CoQ_{10} may be safely used as an alternative to treat hypertension.

Heart Disease Buster

Your heart is the most active muscle in your body. Think about how much it has to work, all the time, day in and day out to bring your cells the energy you need to live. This extreme amount of activity requires a great deal of energy. CoQ_{10} plays a major role in energy production, essential to a healthy heart. It is not surprising then, that while healthy hearts contain high levels of CoQ_{10}, 50 to 75 percent of people with heart disease are deficient in CoQ_{10}. From abundant evidence, gathered over twenty years, the fact that treatment with CoQ_{10} can improve the quality of life and heart function of people with coronary heart disease has been well established.

In one early double-blind trial, CoQ_{10} was given orally to two groups of patients with heart disease. During the course of the study, one group received the supplement first and then a placebo; the other received the placebo first and then the supplement. Levels of CoQ_{10} and heart function were measured at intervals during the study. Both groups experienced increases in cardiac function during the time when they were taking the CoQ_{10}. The patients who had been in steady decline and had not been expected to live more than two years showed great improvement.

In another study, researchers administered CoQ_{10} to nineteen patients who had chronic heart disease. All of the patients began the trial with lower than recommended levels of CoQ_{10} in their blood. After they received the sup - plement, eighteen of the patients reported increased ability to be active. In addition, all patients had improvements in stroke volume, which is a good indicator of heart strength.

Stroke Volume
The amount of blood that the heart pumps out in a single beat.

In yet another early study, 55 percent of patients who received CoQ_{10} in dosages of 30 mg per day for one to two months reported improvements in how they felt, and 30 percent showed a decrease in chest congestion as indicated on X rays. They also had greater stroke volume and cardiac output. The results support the theory that CoQ_{10} can cause the heart muscle to contract with increased force (this is similar to the effect of the widely prescribed heart drug digitalis).

In 1994, a trial in Italy studied 2,664 people with congestive heart failure who were administered daily doses of CoQ_{10} that ranged from 40–150 mg. After three months of treatment, 54 percent of the patients experienced improvement in at least three symptoms that affect quality of life (for example, heart palpitations, shortness of breath, sweating, and fluid retention).

Finally, in one trial, CoQ_{10} was administered to eleven patients who had suffered heart failure and who were potentially eligible for a heart transplant. All those treated with CoQ_{10} showed improvement, with some requiring no further drugs and showing no limit in lifestyle. The authors concluded that the improvement was most likely due to correcting deficiencies of CoQ_{10} in the hearts of these patients, which in turn improved the energy levels in the heart and cardiac performance.

In general, patients with chronic congestive heart failure who have taken CoQ_{10} supplementation are less often hospitalized for worsening of their condition or complications, and show improvements in breathing both at rest and during activity, pulmonary rates, heart rate, palpitation, and blood pressure.

Dosage Recommendations

Usually, the recommended dose of CoQ_{10} ranges from 50–300 mg. Since your body's supply of CoQ_{10} diminishes with age, make sure that you are getting at least 50 mg daily—you may want or need more, depending upon the purpose for which you are taking the coenzyme. Since CoQ_{10} is fat-soluble, your body will absorb it best if it is taken with fatty foods, such as fish. In addition, taking CoQ$_{10}$ in a form (preferably liquid or oil) that contains some vitamin E will help to preserve the coenzyme.

As always, check with your doctor to determine the dosage that is best for you and your unique set of needs.

CHAPTER 8

DHEA

Dyhydroepiandrosterone (DHEA) is a steroid hormone produced primarily in your adrenal glands, which are located just on top of the kidneys. Your body converts DHEA into all other steroid hormones—especially the sexual hormones estrogen and testosterone and cortico-steroids. DHEA is produced in large amounts during youth and young adulthood, but peaks at age twenty, after which time it wanes. By the time you reach age seventy, you may experience a 90 percent reduction in DHEA levels.

Declining levels of DHEA in the body are associated with high cholesterol, heart disease, arthritis, and autoimmune disorders. There has been growing evidence that oral supplementation with DHEA may improve body composition, boost immune function, increase mood and sexual drive, and increase lean body mass and muscle strength. There is also promise for DHEA's ability to improve memory and enhance mental function in older adults, but further research is necessary.

Adrenal Gland
One of a pair of ductless glands, located above the kidneys, which secrete hormones, including DHEA and epinephrine.

Fights Bone Loss

According to one French study, which was cited in the *Harvard Women's Health Newsletter,* healthy women over age seventy who took DHEA had reduced loss of bone, fuller and moister skin, and better complexion. Currently, clinical trials are being conducted in the United States to determine how estrogen and DHEA influence muscle mass, strength, and endurance in women.

Researchers are interested in the potential therapeutic and protective properties of DHEA. In fact, Columbia University's Rosenthal Center for Complementary and Alternative Medicine is conducting a study on DHEA for postmenopausal women who are looking for an alternative to estrogen therapy in order to improve bone density and prevent osteoporosis. The investigators for this study note that postmenopausal women with normal bone density who take DHEA pills experience a strengthening in their bones. This new study seeks to determine whether DHEA supplementation can help women who are past menopause and who already have low bone density.

Enhances Mood and Sex Drive

For a long time, estrogen has been recognized as having an effect on mood in women. The fluctuation of this hormone during a woman's menstrual cycle and during perimenopause (the years of hormonal changes prior to menopause) may lead to feelings of depression and sadness. In addition, DHEA levels have been found to be lower in older women who are clinically depressed. For these reasons, it is thought that supplementation with DHEA can alleviate these symptoms of depression in women. While promising, it is too early to come to a definitive conclusion. There is a large-scale trial currently underway to determine how DHEA affects sex drive, mood, memory, and strength, which soon should shed more light on these questions.

There is some strong evidence of the positive effects of DHEA on the sexual vitality of women. In fact, most clinical trials show some positive effect in women who take DHEA. Researchers at the Boston University School of Medicine evaluated women with different types of sexual dysfunction, including low levels of desire and arousal, and difficulty with orgasm. They found that many of these women had low levels of the male sex hormone testosterone (also known as an androgen). After treating a group of these women with DHEA, the researchers discovered a decrease in sexual distress, an increase in sexual function, and a return to normal values of testosterone. The study's authors concluded that androgen replacement therapy with DHEA seemed to be a safe and effective treatment for female sexual dysfunction. They also noted that more, broader, research is desirable.

To determine the role of DHEA in sexual function, researchers at Harvard Medical School conducted a review of the scientific literature on the subject. They found that increasing DHEA levels in women by a dosage of 50 mg per day leads to greater levels of testosterone and increased sexual thoughts, as well as enhanced moods and feelings of well-being. These observations support the use of DHEA supplements to increase testosterone levels in women to improve sexual satisfaction.

A third clinical study conducted at the University of Washington, Seattle, measured sexual response to an erotic video that was shown to sixteen postmenopausal women who were treated with either oral supplements of DHEA or a placebo one hour before viewing. The investigators found that blood levels of DHEA increased two to five times after receiving the DHEA supplement. In addition, the women who received

DHEA experienced greater mental and physical arousal to the erotic video. This study is yet another showing strong promise for DHEA's effectiveness in enhancing sexual vitality in women.

Improves Body Composition

Clinical Endocrinology reported on the results of the effects of DHEA supplementation on a group of healthy non-obese men and women aged fifty to sixty-five. After receiving 100 mg per day of DHEA for one year, blood levels of DHEA in the people given DHEA supplements were restored to those of young adults. In addition, both men and women experienced an increase in blood levels of insulin-like growth factor, and men showed lowered levels of body fat and increased muscle mass. Researchers speculate that there may be a gender-specific response to DHEA: in other words, its effects may vary in men and women.

Another study at the University of California, San Diego, found that 50 mg a day of DHEA taken for six months resulted in increased lean body mass and muscle strength as well as improved physical and mental well-being in both men and women. However, it is important to note that other well-conducted studies on healthy older adults have not found the increases in muscle mass, or improved sense of well-being, making more study necessary.

Boosts Immune System

It is well known that DHEA boosts the immune system. The hormone is necessary for the development of immune cells and for the production of antibodies. It is believed that DHEA is involved in regulating cytokine production. Cytokines are released by the cells of your immune system, and are similar to hormones, but some cytokines may cause damage. Studies conducted by the University of Tucson in Arizona investigated the effect of DHEA and melatonin in mice with a leukemia retrovirus that leads to AIDS in mice. When administered both DHEA and melatonin, there was an increase in immune cell function, measured by an increase in B and T helper cells, but production of damaging cytokines did not increase.

In addition, as some of us age, we may experience a wasting away of the thymus gland, which is located at the base of the neck and helps to produce our immune system's T cells. This atrophy increases the likelihood of immune dysfunction, which is one of the most destructive effects of aging. DHEA seems to protect the thymus against atrophy caused by stress hormones and therefore can be valuable in preserving the integrity of the immune system.

Dosage Recommendations and Warnings

Although it is available without a prescription in the United States, DHEA is a potent hormone and precursor to estrogen and testosterone. Because DHEA can raise (sometimes in unpredictable ways) estrogen and testosterone levels, it may also increase the risk of cancers of the endometrium, breast, and prostate. The risks simply are not clear, so a hefty dose of caution is warranted. Before taking DHEA, ask your physician to measure your levels of this hormone. Take DHEA only if your levels are below normal, and have followup tests to ensure that you are not taking more than you need to achieve normal levels. If you are under age forty, it is unlikely that you need DHEA.

When DHEA first became popular, many people were taking 50 mg or more daily. Older men often reported having more sexual energy. In women, such dosages sometimes caused acne or facial hair. We now know that such a dosage is excessive for most people who have low DHEA. Smaller dosages, such as 5–15 mg daily—or even three times weekly—may be sufficient for slowly and safely boosting DHEA levels under a physician's supervision.

CHAPTER 9

VITAMINS C AND E

It is helpful to consider vitamin C and vitamin E together when looking at their anti-aging benefits. Each of these vitamins, among the most powerful antioxidants available to us, is obtained through different sources. Vitamin C is found primarily in fruits and vitamin E in vegetables. As antioxidants, vitamins E and C are free-radical scavengers. But while vitamin E scavenges in fatty cell membranes, vitamin C quenches free radicals in watery regions of cells. However, evidence suggests that they work best together (synergistically), meaning that their combined effect is greater than if one or the other is taken alone. Together they provide some of the most important nutritional protection against a large number of diseases and conditions, and can enhance your vitality.

Vitamin C for Immunity and Energy

Nearly everyone is familiar with the healing and health-enhancing powers of vitamin C. The benefits of this powerful antioxidant are myriad: it protects the immune system, fights infections, helps to cure the colds and flu, and increases energy.

The body cannot manufacture vitamin C on its own, so we must get it from our food and from supplements. Vitamin C is water-soluble, and most of the C that you consume is excreted in your urine. Therefore, it must be regularly replaced. It is important not only that our daily diet include foods rich in vitamin C, but also that we take vitamin C supplements.

The best dietary sources of vitamin C are berries, citrus fruits, tomatoes, and raw cabbage.

Vitamin E All Around

Almost as familiar as vitamin C's benefits are the anti-aging benefits of vitamin E. In fact, it may seem like everyone you know is taking large doses of this vitamin. Vitamin E topical creams can be found in every health and beauty store. A widely studied supplement, vitamin E is one of the most potent anti-aging nutrients around. In fact, it has even been referred to as the vitamin equivalent of the "fountain of youth." Vitamin E consists of two groups of molecules: the tocopherols and the tocotrienols. Each of these two groups contains four molecules in alpha, beta, gamma, and delta forms. Of all eight forms of vitamin E, alpha-tocopherol is the most powerful.

Alpha Tocopherol
The most potent of the eight forms of vitamin E.

Along with vitamins A, K, and D, vitamin E is fat-soluble, meaning it is capable of being stored in the body. As an antioxidant, it protects other fat-soluble vitamins, particularly vitamin A, from free-radical destruction. Vitamin E plays an essential role in the circulatory system and is necessary for tissue repair and a host of other bodily functions, including blood clotting and fertility. Too much estrogen, birth control pills, and intake of processed foods can deplete your body of this vital nutrient.

Food sources of vitamin E are dark-green leafy vegetables, nuts, seeds, whole grains, berries, and vegetable oils.

Vitamin E and Exercise-Related Stress

Regular exercise is important. It is good for your body and mind; it can prevent a host of diseases. This you know. But did you also know that the flip side to strenuous exercise is that it also causes some muscular damage. This is because exercise increases oxygen consumption by the body, which leads to an increase of oxygen in the mitochondria, some of which causes oxidative stress and produces potentially damaging free radicals.

This does not mean you should not exercise—the evidence for the benefits of regular activity is just too overwhelming to ignore. Study after study, and the landmark Surgeon General's *Report on Physical Activity and Health* released in 1996, have shown a very strong association between exercise and disease prevention. Furthermore, research indicates that exercise training actually helps to increase your cellular antioxidant defenses. In other words, a trained body becomes quite efficient at limiting the damage that free radicals might do to DNA by increasing antioxidant enzymes.

In an article published by *Nutrition*, Dr. Jeffrey Blumberg and Dr. Jennifer M. Sacheck of the Human Nutrition Research Center on Aging at Tufts University, Boston, discuss the role vitamin E can play when you exercise. Drs. Blumberg and Sacheck point out that although many studies do show that antioxidant enzymes increase with exercise training and thereby offer your body protection against free radicals, it still may be important for exercisers to take higher levels of vitamin E, just to make sure that they have adequate protection. This may be especially true for exercisers who are older; it appears that the older you are, the more susceptible you may be to exercise-induced stress. Also, the harder you train, the more likely it is that you would need extra supplementation.

Vitamin E and Overall Aging

One study of vitamin E that was conducted on middle-aged and older mice at the University of Arizona College of Medicine and the Veterans Affairs Medical Center discovered that age-related damage to proteins in the brain and white blood cells could be prevented or delayed with vitamin E supplementation.

In the study, Dr. Marguerite Kay and her team divided the mice into three groups: one received high levels of vitamin E, one received large doses of beta-carotene (vitamin A), and one received standard amounts of both these nutrients. Seven months later, the mice that received the vitamin E did not have the protein damage typical in aging mice, and their brain tissue functioned more like the tissue in younger mice. "The results suggest that vitamin E, and possibly other antioxidants, may reduce damage associated with aging in the immune and central nervous systems in humans," said Dr. Kay when the results were released in a press release dated May 12, 1996 from the University of Arizona Health Science's Center. She also noted the possibility, as yet unproven, that vitamin E may actually extend life span.

Other studies have found that vitamin E can help to reduce risk of stroke in postmenopausal women, and that the risk of stroke due to blocked arteries (rather than by bleeding in the brain) in male smokers is reduced with vitamin E supplementation.

Vitamins C and E: A Dynamic Duo

Known for their ability to protect against coronary heart disease and other chronic disorders, vitamin E and vitamin C together generally slow the aging process by stabilizing the free radicals in the body. Vitamin E in particular also improves skin tone and prevents age spots, which is why it is such a popular anti-aging cream. It also can prevent exercise-induced cellular damage. Here's a look at some of the evidence of this dynamic duo's effectiveness in improving your health and vitality.

Reduce Overall Risk of Death

Vitamin E and vitamin C may reduce your risk of death from numerous causes, including coronary heart disease. The *American Journal of Clinical Nutrition* published a study conducted by the National Institute on Aging that examined taking supplements of both vitamin E and vitamin C to reduce overall mortality risk. The researchers also were interested in determining whether taking vitamin C along with vitamin E would produce better results than taking vitamin E alone.

The large study looked at more than 11,000 people between ages 67 and 105 who were asked to note all the vitamin supplements, aside from their multivitamin, they were currently taking. By the time the nine-year study was completed, the researchers discovered that those who took vitamin E were 27 percent less likely to have died from any cause, including from coronary heart disease, than those who did not take the supplement. The effects were strongest for protecting against death from heart disease, which produced a 41 percent reduction in death. In addition, those who took both vitamin E and vitamin C supplements had an even greater reduced risk of total mortality and death from heart disease.

The vitamins' ability to stabilize free radicals and therefore prevent the damage that they can do to cells, in particular to the cells that line the arteries, may partly explain these strong protective effects. In addition, both of these vitamins are found abundantly in fruits and vegetables, and consuming large quantities of fruits and vegetables has been proven to lower rates of heart disease, stroke, and cancer.

Cardiovascular Protection

There is more evidence that vitamins C and E can reduce your risk of cardiovascular disease, including heart disease and stroke. Many descriptive controlled studies show a relationship between antioxidant vitamin consumption and reduced risk of cardiovascular disease, and suggest that vitamins C and E may play a role in disease prevention. Treatment with vitamin C has improved the health of blood vessels in patients with coronary artery disease. In addition, older adults who take vitamin C supplements have lower blood pressure than those who don't.

Vitamin E may play a role in keeping your arteries clear. In Italy, researchers conducted a study of 310 middle-aged women who were found to be in the early stages of atherosclerosis (clogging of the arteries). None of the women took vitamin supplements. Their blood plasma levels of vitamins E, C, and A were measured. When the results were analyzed, the researchers found that the women who had lower levels of vitamin E in the blood had greater amounts of artery-clogging plaque. These results suggest that low vitamin E intake can put you at risk for atherosclerosis.

Cancer Protection

Various cancers seem to be protected against by supplementation with vitamins C and E. A report published by the Fred Hutchinson Cancer Research Center in Seattle, Washington, noted that a review of several studies offers insight into the protective effects of these supplements. Specifically, the report cites that randomized clinical trials have shown that vitamin E in the form of alpha-tocopherol can protect against prostate and stomach cancers. Other types of studies have shown that bladder cancer may be related to low levels of vitamin C and that several other cancers, including cancer of the colon, are protected against by vitamin E.

Maintain Brain Power

As we age, some loss of cognitive ability is common. Cognition is the act or process of knowing or perceiving. Cognitive loss related to aging can fall on a continuum: from having slight lapses in memory to full-blown dementia or Alzheimer's disease, in which the ability to reason or remember is severely impaired. People with dementia suffer from a greatly reduced quality of life and are at greater risk of being disabled and of dying. Science has well established that a diet rich in fruits and vegetables can protect brain function and delay the onset of any cognitive impairment.

Because of their strengths as antioxidants and their ability to prevent oxidative damage to brain cells, vitamins E and C are strong frontline protection against future dementia, as well as for treating it in its early stages. In fact, several observational studies support that these vitamins may protect against dementia and Alzheimer's disease.

The journal *Nutrition* reported the results of a study conducted on older adults by researchers in Madrid, Spain. The diets of thirty-four men and eighty-six women between the ages of sixty-five and ninety-one, who showed no signs of significant cognitive impairment, were monitored for five consecutive days. Their blood levels of vitamin E and cholesterol were tested, as was their cognitive ability. Those whose vitamin E intake was below 50 percent of the recommended level had a greater number of errors on the cognitive test. Furthermore, those who had a perfect score on the cognitive test also had higher serum levels of vitamin E. The study showed a clear relationship between vitamin E and cognitive function.

Another study, conducted by the Rush Institute for Healthy Aging and Rush Alzheimer's Disease Center at Rush University in Chicago, examined the use of vitamins E and C and the development of Alzheimer's disease in a prospective study of 633 people who were at least sixty-five years old. (Prospective studies are considered the gold standard by scientists to determine cause and effect.)

Prospective Study

A study carried out on a group over an extended period of time to determine long-term effectiveness of a particular treatment.

After more than four years of study, ninety-one of the participants were diagnosed with Alzheimer's disease. None of the participants who regularly took vitamin E or vitamin C supplements, however, were diagnosed with the disease. In that researchers found that those participants who took only a multivitamin did not receive any protection against Alzheimer's disease, the study's results strongly support supplementation with vitamins E and C to reduce the risk of Alzheimer's disease.

Despite this evidence, we should note that one large prospective study, which was conducted in Japan, found that taking supplements of vitamin E and C did not affect the risk for dementia in the population that was studied. The study, reported in the *Journal of the American Medical Association*, assessed the effectiveness of vitamin E and C supplementation in preventing new cases of dementia. These findings are at odds with the other strong studies that support the efficacy of vitamins E and C in the area of cognition.

Dosage Recommendations

If you smoke or drink alcohol, or take antidepressants and steroids, your levels of vitamin C may be depleted. Some experts recommend taking vitamin C supplements twice each day (just divide your daily dose in half). While considered an extremely safe supplement, excessive intake of vitamin C can cause diarrhea. For most people, 1,000–4,000 mg may be sufficient.

When taking vitamin E supplements, it is best to use a natural source, which your body can better absorb and use. Natural vitamin E is identified on labels as "d-alpha tocopherol (or tocopheryl)," whereas synthetic vitamin E is identified as "dl-alpha tocopherol (or tocopheryl)." A daily dosage of 400 IU of natural vitamin E is beneficial. You might also consider a natural vitamin E supplement that includes other forms of vitamin E called "mixed tocopherols" or "tocotrienols."

Because vitamin E is fat-soluble, it is better to take it along with fish oils and other fats to maximize its absorption and antioxidant protective properties.

CHAPTER 10

HERBS

The medicinal value of many plants is well known. In addition to the vitamins and supplements that we talked about in earlier chapters, several herbs have anti-aging properties. While there is a lot of controversy in the general press about herbal remedies, especially with regard to their potential toxicity and effectiveness, there is strong evidence that when used correctly, herbs are safe and effective natural medicines.

Botanicals have been used by different cultures to both prevent and treat diseases and conditions for centuries. That said, for some herbs or herbal products, there have been cases of unsubstantiated claims of benefits. It's important for you, as a consumer, to be educated and aware. Read up on the herbal treatments that you are considering taking, examine the results of studies as well as the anecdotal history that certain herbs may have in folk medicine. Lastly, always discuss any herbal treatments you are considering with your doctor or primary healthcare practitioner. Together, you can discover if there are any potential negative interactions with other medications you may be taking, and determine the herbal treatments that will best meet your own unique biological needs.

Tips on Using Herbs

It is important to buy brands that are reputable

and that contain pure ingredients. When possible, try to buy herbs that are wildcrafted or organic. Look for standardized extracts of medicinal plants, which means that the product has been analyzed to ensure that it contains consistent levels of key components. For each product, there may be a number of options, including tinctures (alcoholic extracts of plants), freeze-dried extracts, or herbs in capsule form.

Because herbs are very potent—after all they are forms of natural drugs and are not foods or vitamins—take them with the same caution you would a prescription medication. Stop taking an herbal treatment if you notice any kind of allergic reaction. Finally, we all are biologically and emotionally different. So bear in mind that while a particular herb may be good for one person, it may not necessarily be helpful to another. However, it is likely that among the most promising anti-aging herbs, you will find one or more that will benefit you.

Garlic and Ginseng: A Wealth of Benefits

You surely are familiar with garlic as a strong food seasoning. But did you also know that garlic is one of the most potent medicinal herbs around? Garlic has been a popular medicinal herb for centuries, used throughout the world to treat a wide variety of age-related conditions.

In the last decade or so, this powerful anti-oxidant has been studied extensively for its role in preventing or slowing down aging. Its many healthful effects include extending the life span and improving the cognitive function in mice, improving the immune system, protecting against cancer, preventing the formation of cataracts, preventing and treating heart disease, and improving serum cholesterol levels. People eating one fresh clove of garlic a day for sixteen weeks found their cholesterol lowered by 20 percent. In fact, recent studies have shown that garlic, which is a complex herb containing many compounds, has a number of effects on cardiovascular health.

The journal *Circulation* reported the results of a study of garlic's protective effects against heart disease. As you age, your aorta can grow stiff, causing blood not to flow easily. A group of 101 healthy adults age fifty to eighty who were taking 300 mg per day of garlic powder for at least two years were compared with a group of healthy adults who were not taking garlic. After testing both groups, those who took garlic were found to have a more elastic aorta than those who did not take garlic. One or two cloves of garlic a day is the generally recommended dosage.

Aorta
The main artery of the circulation system, which transports blood away from the heart.

Ginseng belongs to the class of herbs known as adaptogens, which are known to fight stress and restore homeostasis in the body. Ginseng comes in several varieties, such as Chinese, Siberian, and American. Its benefits as an anti-aging agent include memory and learning enhancement, immune function improvement, and central nervous system improvement, as well as reduced risk of certain cancers, including gastric and lung cancer.

Ginseng, which improves circulation, also has positive effects on sexual vitality, which can wane with age. It improves libido and has been shown to help men with erectile dysfunction. Ginseng contains an active compound called saponin that is believed to work on the smooth muscle of erectile tissue. Finally, researchers in Japan found that ginseng and du zhong leaf together stimulated the formation of collagen, which normally decreases with age and causes the skin to thin and wrinkle.

Ginkgo Biloba: Protection for Your Mind

What comes to mind when you hear ginkgo? Probably your mind itself. Ginkgo biloba is an antioxidant derived from the ginkgo tree and its leaves have been used for centuries in China as medicinal treatments. Its primary anti-aging benefits are as a memory and general mind en-hancer. It has been shown to have specific effects on cerebral aging by reactivating the noradrenergic system in your brain. Its many effects on brain health include improving memory, learning rate, attention, and con-centration. It even has been effec-tive in treating individuals with Alzheimer's disease.

Noradrenergic Nerve Fibers *Secrete the neurotransmitter noradrenaline.*

A review of four well-conducted scientific studies on the efficacy of ginkgo biloba extract in improving cognitive function of patients with Alz-heimer's disease revealed the following: Three to six months of treatment with 120–240 mg per day of ginkgo biloba extract resulted in improve-ments on objective tests of cognitive function in patients with Alzheimer's disease. In addition, there were no adverse effects from the treatment in any of the clinical trials.

In another study, researchers examined the ability of ginkgo biloba extract to improve the condition of the aging brain. They found that the extract protected brain cells against toxic effects and damage. In addition to its brain-power prop-erties, ginkgo biloba leaves are believed to help improve arteriosclerosis.

Saw Palmetto for Prostate Health

The saw palmetto tree (*Serenoa repens*) is indig -

enous to Florida. This fruit-bearing palm tree is particularly helpful to men with benign prostatic hyperplasia (BPH). BPH is a common, nonmalignant enlargement of the prostate gland that will affect more than half of all men at some point in their lives (usually after age fifty). It is caused by the androgen, estrogen, and pituitary hormonal changes that occur in the body as men age. Although it is not life threatening, BPH can lead to urinary tract problems. In particular, it can ob - struct the bladder, causing an increased urge to urinate and awakenings during the night. It also can interfere with the flow of urine, slowing it down.

Several well-conducted scientific clinical trials have tested the effectiveness of saw palmetto in treating BPH. An analysis of these trials shows that when compared with placebo treatment, saw palmetto improves the symptoms of BPH as well as normalizes urine flow. Patients also experienced only mild side effects, such as headache or upset stomach, and these were only in - frequently reported.

The herbs presented in this chapter are just a few of the major herbs that have been effective in preventing or delaying some of the conditions associated with aging. Others that you may want to investigate include aloe, licorice, evening primrose oil, and valerian. Aloe has great ability to restore damaged tissues; licorice seems to help patients with diabetes; evening primrose oil helps patients with rheumatoid arthritis and may also lower blood pressure and cholesterol; and valerian has been widely used as a sleep aid for thousands of years.

CONCLUSION

None of us can avoid growing older. It is a fact of life. We live; we age. However, we can dramatically slow down and, in some cases, reverse the effects of aging.

Aging can be attacked on several fronts. First, there is the issue of lifestyle, which includes diet, activity level, and habits. These areas all involve choices we make—some consciously, others maybe without thinking—that can have a huge impact on how well we age. By eating a diet that is rich in nutrients, ensuring that we get enough exercise, and avoiding negative habits such as smoking, excessive alcohol drinking, and sun bathing without protection, we can erase years from our age. The great thing about lifestyle is that ultimately it is all up to us. We have the power to effect great positive results by making some changes.

Many scientists believe that oxidative stress and the damage caused by free radicals is responsible for most of the effects of aging. Free radicals work at a cellular level to gradually chip away at our youth and vitality; their effect is cumulative. Antioxidants, often referred to as free-radical scavengers, help keep free radicals in check. Through their ability to combat the damage of free radicals, they can help us to avoid both the chronic diseases and poor skin conditions associated with aging. There is increasing evidence and acceptance in the scientific community of the protective effects of antioxidant supplementation on aging. This book presented information about several antioxidants that can help keep you younger and healthy.

Antioxidants aren't the only line of defense we have against aging. We also saw that several hormones, amino acids, vitamins, minerals, and herbs can have a positive effect on aging. Each works through specific mechanisms to address particular aging issues. All of the supplements discussed in this book are strong, powerful, and effective. However, they may affect different people differently, depending on a variety of factors. Before you take supplements, always consult with a healthcare practitioner to make sure you are making the choices that are best for you.

In the end, aging comes down to energy. The more energy our bodies have at the cellular level, the more energy we will have to live our lives the way we want to, and the younger we will look and feel. The nutrients discussed in this book all may help our bodies to increase energy and offer protection against common age-related diseases and conditions. The most important thing is to remain independent, healthy, and vital for as long as we can. There is every reason to believe that while we may be older by virtue of years, we can enjoy life the way we did when we were younger— with that same kind of enthusiasm, energy, and positive outlook. In so doing, perhaps we can, in fact, be "forever" young.

SELECTED
REFERENCES

Breithaupt-Grogler K, Ling M, Boudoulas H, et al. Protective effect of chronic garlic intake on elastic properties of aorta in the elderly. *Circulation*, 1997; 96(8): 2649–2655.

Buckley LM, Hillner BE. A cost effectiveness analysis of calcium and vitamin D supplementation, etidronate, and alendronate in the prevention of vertebral fractures in women treated with glucocorticoids. *Journal of Rheumatology*, 2003; 30(1): 132–138.

Carta A, Calvani M, Bravi D, et al. Acetyl-L-carnitine and Alzheimer's disease: pharmacological considerations beyond the cholinergic sphere. *Annals of New York Academy of Sciences*, 1993; 695: 324–326

Dvorkin L, Song KY. Herbs for benign prostatic hyperplasia. *Annals of Pharmacotherapy*, 2002; 36(9): 1443–1452.

Ervin RB, Kennedy-Stephenson J. Mineral intakes of elderly adult supplement and non-supplement users in the third national health and nutrition examination survey. *Nutrition*, 2002; 132(11): 3422–3427.

Goodwin JS, Goodwin JM, Garry PJ. Association between nutritional status and cognitive functioning in a healthy elderly population. *Journal of the American Medical Association*, 1983; 249(21): 2917–2921.

Hagen Tm, Liu J, Lukkesfeldt J, et al. Feeding acetyl-L-carnitine and lipoic acid to old rats significantly improves metabolic function while decreasing oxidative stress. *Proceedings of the National Academy of Sciences of the USA*, 2002; 99: 1870–1875.

Holt PR, Atillasoy EO, Gilman J, et al. Modulation of abnormal colonic epithelial cell proliferation and differentiation by low-fat dairy foods: a randomized controlled trial. *Journal of the American Medical Association*, 1998; 280(12): 1074–1079.

Iannuzzi A, Celentano E, Panico S, et al. Dietary and circulating antioxidant vitamins in relation to carotid plaques in middle-aged women. *American Journal of Clinical Nutrition*, 2002; 76(3): 582–587.

Lenhart SE, Nappi JM. Vitamins for the management of cardiovascular disease: a simple solution to a complex problem? *Pharmacotherapy*, 1999; 19(12): 1200–1212.

Lockwood K, Moesgaard S, Hanioka T, et al. Apparent partial remission of breast cancer in 'high risk' patients supplemented with nutrition antioxidants, essential fatty acids and coenzyme Q10. *Molecular Aspects of Medicine*, 1994; 15: Suppl p. 231–240.

Losonczy KG, Harris TB, Havlik RJ. Vitamin E and vitamin C supplement use and risk of all-cause and coronary heart disease mortality in older persons: the established populations for epidemiologic studies of the elderly. *American Journal of Clinical Nutrition*, 1996; 64(2): 190–196.

Morales AJ, Haubrich RH, Hwang JY et al. The effect of six months treatment with a 100 mg dose of dehydroepiandrosterone (dhea) on circulating sex steroids, body composition and muscle strength in age-advanced men and women. *Clinical Endocrinology,* 1998; 49(4): 421–432.

Munarriz R, Talakoub L, Flaherty E, et al. Androgen replacement therapy with dehydroepiandrosterone for androgen insufficiency and female sexual dysfunction: androgen and questionnaire results. *Journal of Sex and Marital Therapy,* 2002; 28 Suppl 1: 165–173.

Nourhashemi, F, Gillette-Guyonnet S, Andrieu S, et al. Alzheimer's disease: protective factors. *American Journal of Clinical Nutrition,* 2000; 71(2): 643S-649S.

Pereria MA, Krska AM, Day RD, et al. A randomized walking trial in postmenopausal women. *Archives of Internal Medicine,* 1998; 158 (15): 1695–1701.

Riggs KM, Spiro A, Tucker K et al. Relations of vitamin B-12, vitamin B-6, folate, and homocysteine to cognitive performance in the normative aging study. *American Journal of Clinical Nutrition,* 1996; 63(3): 306–314.

Sacheck JM, Blumberg JB. Role of vitamin E and oxidative stress in exercise. *Nutrition,* 2001; 17(10): 809–814.

Seshadri S, Beiser A, Selhub J, et al. Plasma homocysteine as a risk factor for dementia and Alzheimer's disease. *The New England Journal of Medicine,* 2002; 346: 476–483.

Shults CW, Oakes D, Kieburtz K et al. Effects of coenzyme Q10 in early Parkinson disease: evidence of slowing of the functional decline. *Archives of Neurology,* 2002; 59(10): 1541–1550.

Stewart KJ. Exercise training and the cardio-vascular consequences of type 2 diabetes and hypertension. *Journal of the American Medical Association,* 2002; 288(13): 1622–1631.

Yoshida S, Honda A, Matsuzaki Y, et al. Anti-proliferative action of endogenous dehydroepiandrosterone metabolites on human cancer cell lines. *Steroids*, 2003; 68(1): 73–83.

Zhdanova IV, Wurtman RJ, Regan MM et al. Melatonin treatment for age-related insomnia. *Journal of Clinical Endocrinology & Metabolism*, 2001; 86(10): 4727–4730.

OTHER BOOKS
AND RESOURCES

Barney P. *Doctor's Guide to Natural Medicine*, Pleasant Grove, Utah: Woodland Publishing Inc., 1998.

Challem J, Berkson B, and Smith MD. *Syndrome X: The Complete Nutritional Guide to Preventing and Reversing Insulin Resistance.* New York, John Wiley & Sons, 2000.

Challem J and Brown L. *User's Guide to Vitamins and Minerals*, North Bergen, New Jersey: Basic Health Publications, 2002.

Daniels D. *Exercises for Osteoporosis*, Long Island City, New York: Hatherleigh Press, 2000.

Fuchs, N. *User's Guide to Calcium and Magnesium*, North Bergen, New Jersey: Basic Health Publications, 2002.

GreatLife Magazine
Consumer magazine with articles on vitamins, minerals, herbs, and foods.
Available for free at many health and natural food stores.

Let's Live Magazine
Consumer magazine with emphasis on the health benefits of vitamins, minerals, and herbs.

Customer service:
1-800-676-4333

P.O. Box 74908

Los Angeles, CA 90004

Subscriptions: 12 issues per year, $19.95 in the U.S.; $31.95 outside the U.S.

Physical Magazine

Magazine oriented to body builders and other serious athletes.

Customer service:

1-800-676-4333

P.O. Box 74908

Los Angeles, CA 90004

Subscriptions: 12 issues per year, $19.95 in the U.S.; $31.95 outside the U.S.

The Nutrition Reporter™ newsletter

Monthly newsletter that summarizes recent medical research on vitamins, minerals, and herbs.

Customer service:

P.O. Box 30246

Tucson, AZ 85751-0246

e-mail: jack@thenutritionreporter.com

www.nutritionreporter.com

Subscriptions: $26 per year (12 issues) in the U.S.; $32 U.S. or $48 CNC for Canada; $38 for other countries.

INDEX

Printed in the USA
CPSIA information can be obtained
at www.ICGtesting.com
JSHW012007140824
68134JS00004B/47

9 781681 628394